NAHID PERVEEN

BRIDGING THE GAP BETWEEN modern science AND ayurveda FOR HEALTHY AND ENERGETIC LIVING

GUT/IMMUNITY/MARMA/SKIN& SENSES/HAIR

BlueRose ONE.com
Stories Matter
NewDelhi • London

BLUEROSE PUBLISHERS
India | U.K.

For permissions requests or inquiries regarding this publication, please contact:

BLUEROSE PUBLISHERS
www.BlueRoseONE.com
info@bluerosepublishers.com
+91 8882 898 898
+4407342408967

ISBN: 978-93-5989-872-8

Cover design: Tahira
Typesetting: Tanya Raj Upadhyay

First Edition: April 2024

Secret of
Ayurveda or
holistic healing of gut
and
overall health

Table of Contents

Modern era health issues

As urbanisation spread like fire 🔥 same as tension, depression, chronic disease, neuroinflammation, Agni/transformational energy imbalance (mitochondrial dysfunction) also start spreading in our new generation as

Kapha_Bala/ strength, immunity/ ojas, In Ayurveda, Kapha Bala refers to the strength of the Kapha dosha, which is responsible for our immunity and overall stability. It plays a vital role in maintaining a strong immune system and keeping us healthy. Kapha Bala is associated with qualities like endurance, resilience, and the ability to fight off diseases. It's important to balance the Kapha dosha to maintain optimal health and well-being.

• So many young kids development lifestyle disorder like sinusitis (mucus/excess kapha obstruction in nasal passages) and due to weak tissues of lungs mucus form by body just to protect itself from collapsing, it's a way of self defence by our body also due to toxin build in body leads to weak tissues.

Note: that's why ayurveda mostly focus on prevention

White foods like sugar, dairy, and processed grains are often avoided in asthma because they can trigger inflammation and mucus production in the airways, making breathing more difficult. It's best to focus on a diet rich in fruits, vegetables, and whole grains for better respiratory health , Absolutely! There are several remedies in Ayurveda to strengthen Kapha Bala. Here are a few suggestions:

1. Follow a Kapha-balancing diet: Include warm, light, and easily digestible foods in your diet. Opt for spices like ginger, black pepper, and cinnamon. Avoid heavy, oily, and cold foods.
2. Engage in regular exercise: Stay active to stimulate your metabolism and promote circulation. Choose activities that are invigorating and energizing, such as brisk walking, yoga, or dancing.
3. Maintain a regular sleep schedule: Getting enough sleep is crucial for balancing Kapha. Aim for 7-8 hours of quality sleep each night and establish a consistent sleep routine.
4. Practice deep breathing: Deep breathing exercises like pranayama can help balance Kapha and enhance vitality. Try alternate nostril breathing or Kapalabhati breathing.
5. Stay hydrated: Drink warm water throughout the day to keep your body hydrated and support the elimination of toxins.

Note _ white food like sugar diary processed grain is acidic in nature it should be consumed in moderation for everyone.

• apart from lifestyle disorder mucus(excess kapha)forms and causes obstruction in almost all disease including AIDS, excess kapha or mucus sometimes form in body just to protect itself but also have negetive impact on body like congestion, heavyness etc, According to Ayurveda, an imbalance in Kapha dosha can lead to the accumulation of mucus or "vikrut kapha." This can manifest as excess phlegm, congestion, or a feeling of heaviness in the body. To address this imbalance, Ayurveda recommends incorporating lifestyle and dietary practices that help balance Kapha, such as consuming warm, light, and easily digestible foods, staying hydrated, and engaging in regular physical activity. Additionally, herbal remedies like ginger, turmeric, and licorice can be beneficial in reducing mucus and promoting healthy respiratory function.

2. Oleation therapy and hydration

In Ayurveda Mucus is Vikrut kapha or imbalance in kapha/excess kapha _Mucus is mala(waste product of body) and kapha in balance is Bala (strength) and immunity (ojas)

Ghee is known for its amazing properties in Ayurveda. It can help balance Pitta and Vata doshas, which is great for maintaining overall harmony in the body. Ghee is also beneficial for promoting healthy rasa (body fluids), sukr (reproductive tissues), and ojas (vitality). It has a soothing effect and can help alleviate burning sensations. Additionally, ghee is believed to make the body soft, improve the quality of voice, and enhance complexion. It's important to choose good-quality ghee for maximum benefits. It's fascinating how natural ingredients can have such positive effects on our well-being,

Oleation therapy internal good medicated ghee or oil or good fat consumption prescribed in condition like vata diesease, drying kind of body, planning for detox therapy, who exercise daily, consume alcohol daily, who engage in intercourse frequently and also get stressed out easily

In Ayurveda, Sneha, or fats of vegetable origin, like tisi(linseed /flaxseed), walnut, radish, pistachio, and sahijan, are valued for their nourishing and balancing properties. These fats are believed to support various bodily functions these fats are great for promoting healthy skin, supporting digestion, and providing essential fatty acids and are often used in Ayurvedic cooking and medicinal preparations. They are considered to be beneficial for overall wellness

Note: in case of allergy related issues oleation or abhyanga on chest and back is good thing to include in routine,Massaging the chest and back with abhayanga can improve lung capacity and respiratory function

In cases of moderate doshas or mild diseases, a moderate or low dose of ghee, around 15-20ml, may be prescribed to help alleviate the symptoms. This can be beneficial for individuals who are older, younger, or lead a luxurious lifestyle, as well as those with a weak digestive fire. Low dose of Ghee can also be helpful for people who have been suffering from long-term fever, cough, or low strength. Additionally, it can provide relief for those who experience difficulty after gut evacuation.

Ghee, especially medicated ghee, is considered excellent for boosting ojas and immunity. It is believed to nourish and strengthen the body, promoting overall well-being. The rich nutrients and natural properties of ghee are thought to support the immune system and enhance vitality. Including ghee in your diet, in moderation, can be a wonderful way to support your body's natural defenses and maintain a healthy immune system. It's amazing how something as simple as ghee can have such powerful benefits!

When your body is in a hydrated and alkaline state, it creates an optimal environment for repair and healing. Adequate hydration helps to flush out toxins and support various bodily functions. An alkaline environment can help reduce inflammation and promote cellular repair. Together, these conditions provide your body with the surplus of energy it needs to focus on repairing tissues, organs, and overall wellbeing. So, staying hydrated and consuming alkaline-rich foods can contribute to your body's natural repair processes. Cheers to a healthy and balanced lifestyle!

The human body is truly remarkable in its ability to heal and repair itself. In certain cases, such as bone fractures, the body can regenerate and regrow new bone tissue. When it comes to wasting muscle or organ damage, creating a hydrated and alkaline environment can indeed support the body's natural repair processes. By staying hydrated and maintaining a balanced pH level, we can provide the optimal conditions for our body to heal and rejuvenate. It's incredible how our body works to restore itself and promote overall well-being. Taking care of ourselves through proper hydration and a healthy lifestyle can greatly contribute to this amazing healing capacity.

Radish and imli (tamarind) are considered alkalizing in Ayurveda and can have beneficial effects on various abdominal problems. They contain natural alkaline compounds, which can help in managing issues like anorexia, indigestion, constipation, and even certain gastrointestinal conditions like stones, parasites, and fistula. Additionally, the use of Swet Parpati, an Ayurvedic herbal formulation, is known for its alkaline properties and is often used to support digestive health.

Water plays a crucial role in our overall health. Since our bodies are made up of about 60-80% water, staying properly hydrated is essential for maintaining optimal health. Water is involved in countless bodily functions, including regulating body temperature, aiding digestion, transporting nutrients, lubricating joints, and flushing out toxins. By ensuring we're adequately hydrated, we can make a significant difference in our overall well-being. So let's raise a glass to staying hydrated and taking care of our health!

While breath work alone may not directly create an alkaline environment in the body, certain breathing techniques can promote relaxation and reduce stress. This can directly support overall alkalinity by reducing the production of acidforming hormones. Deep, slow breaths, focusing on exhaling fully, can help activate the parasympathetic nervous system, which promotes a sense of calm and balance in the body. Pairing breath work with other lifestyle factors like a healthy diet and regular exercise can contribute to a more alkalinefriendly environment. So, while it may not directly create alkalinity, breath work can still have positive effects on our overall well-being. Breathe deep and feel the calm!

Radish is indeed considered important in Ayurveda and acts as an alkalizing agent. It has a "kahar" or alkaline effect on the body, which can help balance acidity and promote overall well-being. Radishes are known for their digestive properties and can help stimulate digestion. They are also rich in nutrients like Vitamin C and potassium. Including radishes in your diet can be a great way to support your health.

Incorporating radish pickle into your diet is super easy. Here's a simple way to do it:

1. Get fresh radishes and wash them thoroughly.
2. Cut the radishes into thin slices or small cubes.
3. In a clean, dry jar, layer the radish slices and sprinkle some salt between each layer.
4. Add some spices like mustard seeds, cumin seeds, or red chili flakes for extra flavor, if you like.
5. Squeeze some lemon juice over the radishes for a tangy twist.

6. Close the jar tightly and let it sit at room temperature for a day or two to allow fermentation to occur.
7. Once ready, your radish pickle is good to go!

You can enjoy radish pickle as a side dish with your meals, or add it to sandwiches, wraps, or salads for an extra zing. It's a delicious way to incorporate radishes into your diet and reap their health benefits.

Alkaline water is said to help neutralize acid in the bloodstream, boost metabolism, and slow bone loss.

Cucumber infused water is not only refreshing, but it also helps in hydrating the body and provides the benefits of alkaline water. It's a delicious and healthy way to stay hydrated.

Resolution to internal conflict

As per research in modern time psychosomatic diesease are prevailing.

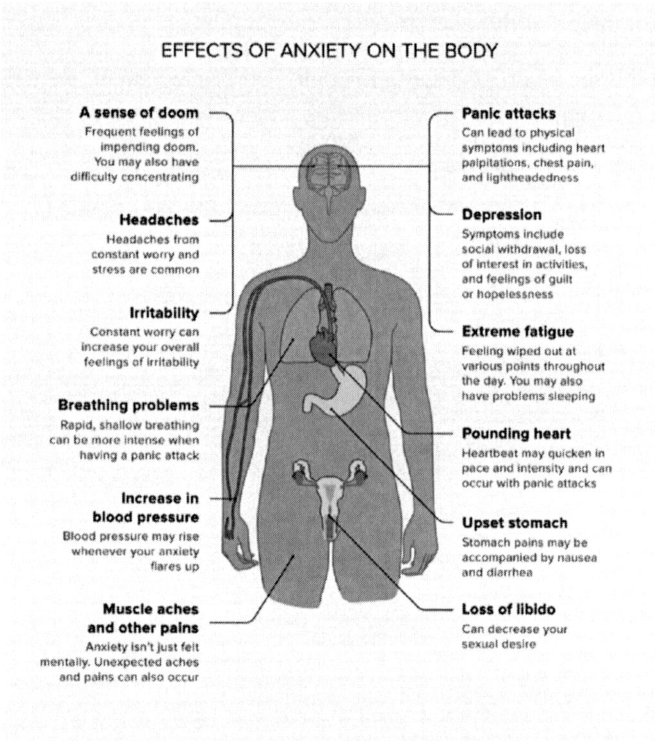

Psychosomatic diseases are conditions in which emotional or mental factors play a significant role in causing or worsening physical symptoms. These symptoms can include pain, fatigue, digestive issues, skin problems, and more. The mind-body connection is important in understanding and managing these diseases, as addressing the underlying psychological factors can help alleviate the physical symptoms. It's a fascinating field that highlights the intricate relationship between our thoughts, emotions, and physical well-being.Low vagal tone can have various causes. It can be due to chronic stress, lack of physical activity, inflammation, or certain medical conditions. It's important to address these factors to improve vagal tone.

low vagal tone can definitely mess with gut permeability. When the vagus nerve isn't functioning optimally, it can lead to increased intestinal permeability, also known as "leaky gut." This means that the lining of the intestines becomes more permeable, allowing harmful substances to pass through and trigger an immune response. It's important to support vagal tone to maintain a healthy gut!

When vagal tone is low, it can have several consequences on the body. It may lead to digestive issues, such as poor digestion and constipation. It can also affect heart health, causing irregular heart rhythms and difficulty regulating blood pressure. Additionally, low vagal tone is associated with increased inflammation and impaired immune function. It's important to take steps to improve vagal tone for overall well-being.

With constant fear and anxiety develop Autoimmune conditions like psoriasis etc, there is evidence to suggest that psychological factors can influence the development and progression of autoimmune conditions. Chronic stress, including fear and anxiety, can potentially trigger or exacerbate autoimmune responses by affecting the immune system and increasing inflammation in the body Internal conflict can be compared to an autoimmune disease in the sense that both involve the body turning against itself. In the case of autoimmune diseases, the immune system mistakenly attacks healthy cells and tissues. Similarly, internal conflict refers to the turmoil and struggle that occurs within a person's mind or emotions. It's like a battle between different thoughts, feelings, or desires, where one part of you may be at odds with another part. Just as autoimmune diseases can cause harm to the body, internal conflict can also have negative impacts on one's well-being and overall harmony. It's important to address and find resolution to internal conflicts in order to promote inner peace and emotional wellbeing. However, it's important to note that autoimmune diseases are complex and multifactorial, with genetic, environmental, and other factors also playing a role. Managing stress and promoting emotional well-being through techniques like relaxation exercises, mindfulness.

Internal conflict can have a profound impact on our overall well-being, including our physical health. When we experience chronic internal conflict, it can lead to prolonged stress and emotional distress. This chronic stress can trigger physiological responses in the body, such as an increase in stress hormones like cortisol, which can negatively affect our immune system and other bodily functions. Over time, this can contribute to the development or exacerbation of chronic diseases, including autoimmune diseases. It's important to address and manage internal conflicts to reduce stress and promote a healthier mind-body balance. Taking care of our mental and emotional well-being is crucial for maintaining overall health and preventing the onset of chronic diseases.

To avoid internal conflict, it can be helpful to practice selfreflection and self-awareness. Take the time to understand your values, beliefs, and priorities. This can help you make decisions that align with your true self and reduce inner turmoil. It's also important to communicate openly and honestly with yourself and others. Expressing your thoughts and feelings can prevent misunderstandings and potential conflicts. Additionally, finding healthy outlets for stress, such as exercise, meditation, or creative activities, can help manage emotions and promote inner peace. Remember, it's okay to seek support from trusted friends, family, or professionals if you need assistance in navigating internal conflicts.

Managing internal conflict can be beneficial for overall wellbeing, including reducing the risk of developing autoimmune diseases. When it comes to managing internal conflict, it's important to prioritize self-care and stress management. This can include activities like practicing mindfulness, engaging in regular exercise, getting enough sleep, and maintaining a balanced diet. Additionally, seeking support from loved ones or professionals, such as therapists or counselors, can provide guidance and help in navigating internal conflicts. Remember, taking care of your mental and emotional health is essential for maintaining a healthy body and reducing the risk of various health conditions, including autoimmune diseases.

Conflict can definitely happen when people don't understand each other's intentions. It's important to make sure we're on the same page and communicate openly to avoid misunderstandings.

Conflict can often arise when there's a disconnect between understanding and intentions. It's like speaking different languages without a translator. Clear communication and mutual understanding are key to resolving conflicts. Conflict can definitely arise when there's a mismatch between understanding and intentions. It's important to communicate clearly and make sure everyone is on the same page.

Good communication truly occurs when our intentions and understanding are in harmony. When we express ourselves clearly and listen actively, we create a space for mutual understanding to flourish. It's all about aligning our intentions with our words and making sure that we understand each other's perspectives. By fostering open and honest communication, we can build stronger connections and resolve conflicts more effectively. So let's keep striving for that harmonious balance in our communication! Good communication is indeed important to avoid conflicts. When we communicate effectively, we can prevent misunderstandings, clarify our intentions, and address any potential issues before they escalate into conflicts. By actively listening, expressing ourselves clearly, and seeking mutual understanding, we can foster healthy and harmonious relationships. So let's keep prioritizing good communication to create a peaceful and conflict-free environment!

Thinking aloud is not only a helpful method for ordering our thoughts and improving concentration, but there are scientific reasons behind it as well. When we vocalize our thoughts, it engages multiple parts of our brain involved in language processing and working memory. This can enhance our cognitive abilities, including problem-solving and decision-making. Additionally, speaking out loud can help us externalize our thoughts, making them more tangible and easier to analyze. So, thinking aloud combines the power of language and cognition to boost our mental processes. It's pretty fascinating, Thinking aloud is an excellent method for ordering our thoughts and improving concentration. When we speak out loud, it helps us organize our ideas and stay focused on the task at hand. It's like having a conversation with ourselves, allowing us to clarify our thoughts and make connections more easily. So the next time you need to concentrate or gather your thoughts, give thinking aloud a try!

Maintaining vagal tone can be accomplished through various practices. Deep breathing exercises, such as diaphragmatic breathing, can help stimulate the vagus nerve. Engaging in activities like yoga, meditation, or tai chi can also have a positive impact on vagal tone. Regular physical exercise, stress reduction techniques, and getting enough sleep are other important factors. Additionally, incorporating healthy lifestyle habits like a balanced diet and avoiding excessive alcohol consumption can contribute to maintaining vagal tone.

Diaphragmatic breathing, also known as belly breathing, is a technique where you focus on breathing deeply into your belly rather than shallowly into your chest. It helps to activate the diaphragm muscle, which in turn stimulates the vagus nerve. To practice diaphragmatic breathing, sit or lie down in a comfortable position. Place one hand on your chest and the other on your abdomen. Take a slow, deep breath in through your nose, letting your belly rise as you fill your lungs with air. Exhale slowly through your mouth, feeling your belly lower. Repeat this process, focusing on the sensation of your breath in your abdomen. It's a simple yet effective way to promote relaxation and improve vagal tone. Give it a try!

So the more we start getting closer to nature fresh air, water and at the same time sorround yourself with good people or friends, who helps you in getting a better person and grow together in all parts of our life, especially in teenagers they seek for love and care and end up with making wrong friends which is the triggering factor for their emotional and mental health,

The vagus nerve is indeed connected to the 4th quadrant of the ear. The auricular branch of the vagus nerve travels to the ear, specifically the cymba conchae, which is a part of the 4th quadrant. Stimulating this area through techniques like auricular acupuncture or auriculotherapy can have an impact on vagal tone and overall well-being. It's fascinating how different parts of our body are interconnected,

- The connection between the ear and the vagus nerve is through the auricular branch of the vagus nerve, which runs through the ear. Stimulating this branch can have an indirect impact on the gut, as the vagus nerve plays a crucial role in regulating digestive functions.
- There are a few ways you can stimulate the vagus nerve through the ear in your daily routine. One method is auricular acupuncture, where small needles are placed on specific points of the ear to activate the nerve. Another technique is using ear seeds or ear magnets, which are small adhesive devices placed on specific points of the ear to provide continuous stimulation.
- If you're interested in exploring these techniques further, I recommend consulting with a qualified acupuncturist or auriculotherapy practitioner who can guide you through the process and find the most suitable points for your needs. It's amazing how such a small part of our

body can have such a big impact on our overall well-being!

- massaging the ear can be a simple and effective way to stimulate the vagus nerve. You can gently massage the outer ear, including the earlobe and the surrounding areas. Use your fingertips to apply gentle pressure and make circular motions. You can also try pulling on the earlobe gently.

This can help activate the auricular branch of the vagus nerve, which runs through the ear. By stimulating this nerve, you may experience relaxation, stress relief, and improved digestion. It's a soothing and easy technique you can incorporate into your daily routine. Give it a try and see how it makes you feel.

"tapping therapy" or Emotional Freedom Technique (EFT). It's a practice where you tap on certain points on your body while focusing on specific emotions or issues. Some people find it helpful to do it in the morning as a way to start their day on a positive note. It can be a great way to release stress and promote emotional well-being.

specific tapping points used in tapping therapy. The basic tapping points are:

1. Top of the head: Tap gently with your fingertips on the crown of your head.
2. Eyebrow: Tap on the inner end of your eyebrow, near the bridge of your nose.
3. Side of the eye: Tap on the outer corner of your eye, on the bone.
4. Under the eye: Tap on the bone just below your eye, in line with your pupil.

5. Under the nose: Tap on the area between your nose and upper lip.
6. Chin: Tap on the middle of your chin, just below your lower lip.
7. Collarbone: Tap on the junction where your collarbone meets the breastbone.
8. Under the arm: Tap on the side of your body, about 4 inches below your armpit.

Remember to tap gently on each point, using your fingertips, while focusing on the specific issue or emotion you want to address.

Tapping therapy, or Emotional Freedom Technique (EFT), is primarily used for emotional and psychological well-being. While it may help reduce stress and promote relaxation

Ah, I see you're interested in using tapping therapy to reduce dark circles. While tapping therapy is primarily used for emotional well-being, it may indirectly help with dark circles by reducing stress and promoting relaxation. Dark circles can sometimes be caused by stress and lack of sleep, so by addressing those factors through tapping therapy, you may see some improvement. However, it's important to note that individual results may vary. It's always a good idea to also incorporate other skincare practices, such as getting enough sleep, staying hydrated.

Note:Tapping the shoulder with fingers after a severe accident or emergency case can serve as a way to check for responsiveness. It's a gentle stimulus that can help assess if the person is conscious or in need of immediate medical attention. Emergency responders often use this technique to gauge a person's level of consciousness and determine the appropriate course of action. It's important to remember that in such situations, it's crucial to seek professional medical help as soon as possible.

Abhyanga is a traditional Ayurvedic practice that involves a full-body massage using warm oil. The word "Abhyanga" itself means "oil massage" in Sanskrit. It's a deeply relaxing and rejuvenating experience that aims to balance the mind, body, and spirit. The massage typically involves long, flowing strokes, rhythmic movements, and gentle pressure applied to different parts of the body. The warm oil used in Abhyanga helps nourish the skin, promote circulation, and release tension. It's a wonderful way to pamper yourself daily before bath and promote overall well-being. Let me know if you have any more questions or if there's anything else I can assist you with! some steps for a selflymphatic massage. Here's a simple routine you can try:

1. Find a comfortable position: Sit or lie down in a relaxed position, ensuring that you have enough space to move your hands freely.
2. Start with neck and face: Gently place your hands on the sides of your neck and use light, upward strokes towards your ears. Then, move to your face and use small, circular motions around your cheeks, temples, and forehead.
3. Move to the armpits: Place your hands in your armpits and gently massage in small circles. This area has many lymph nodes, so spend a little more time here.
4. Work on the chest: Use gentle, upward strokes from the middle of your chest towards your collarbones. You can also use light tapping motions in this area.

5. Focus on the abdomen: With gentle clockwise circular motions, massage your abdomen. This can help stimulate lymphatic flow in the abdominal area.
6. Move to the limbs: Use long, upward strokes on your arms and legs, starting from the hands and feet and moving towards the armpits and groin area.
7. Finish with the back: If you can reach, use long, upward strokes on your back, starting from the lower back and moving towards the upper back.

Abhayanga, along with lymphatic massage, offers a range of benefits for your overall wellbeing. Here are some of the benefits:

1. Relaxation: Abhayanga and lymphatic massage can help promote deep relaxation by reducing stress and anxiety. The rhythmic strokes and gentle pressure help calm the nervous system.
2. Improved circulation: The massage techniques used in Abhayanga and lymphatic massage can enhance blood circulation, which helps deliver oxygen and nutrients to the cells, promoting overall health.
3. Detoxification: Lymphatic massage specifically targets the lymphatic system, which plays a vital role in removing toxins and waste from the body. By stimulating lymphatic flow, it supports the body's natural detoxification process.
4. Enhanced immune function: The lymphatic system is closely linked to the immune system. By improving lymphatic flow, Abhayanga and lymphatic massage can help strengthen the immune system, supporting better overall health.
5. Nourished skin: The use of warm oil in

Abhayanga helps nourish and moisturize the skin, leaving it soft, supple, and glowing. It can also help improve the appearance of dry or rough skin.

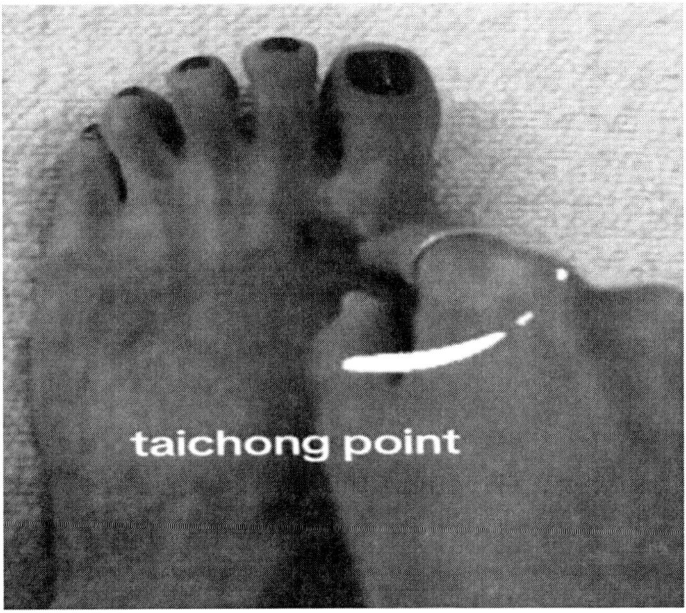

6. Improved digestion: Abhayanga and lymphatic massage can aid in digestion by stimulating the abdominal area and

The Taichong point, also known as Liver 3, is an acupuncture point located on the foot. It's believed to have various benefits, such as promoting liver health, relieving stress, and improving overall well-being. Acupuncture practitioners often use this point to address issues related to the liver and emotional well-being. It's fascinating how acupuncture can have such a positive impact on our bodies and minds!

here are some general common points in both abhyanga and lymphatic massage

1. Choose the right oil: Select a highquality oil that suits your dosha (body type) or the specific needs of your skin and body. Common oils used in Abhyanga include sesame oil, coconut oil, and almond oil.
2. Warm the oil: Gently warm the oil by placing the bottle in a bowl of warm water. Avoid overheating the oil as it can cause burns.

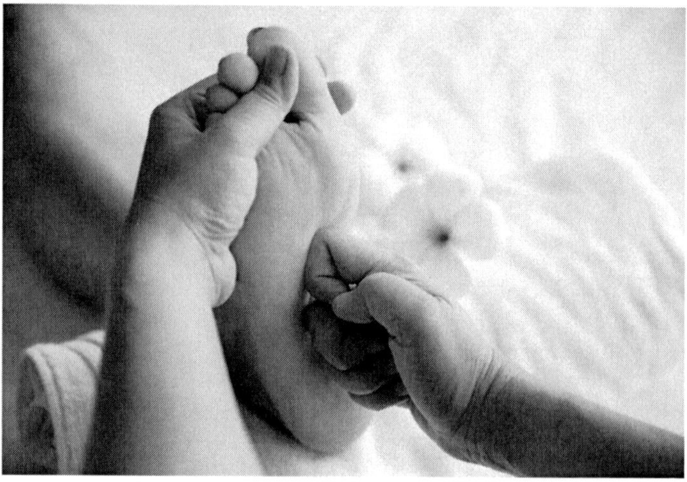

3. Create a calm environment: Find a quiet and comfortable space where you can relax and enjoy the massage.
   While a foot massage before bed may not directly impact eye health, it can definitely contribute to overall relaxation and well-being, which can indirectly benefit your eyes. When you're relaxed and stress-free, it can help reduce eye strain and promote better sleep, which is essential for maintaining healthy eyes. So go ahead and enjoy your foot massage for a good night's rest.
4. Start with self-massage: Begin by applying a small amount of warm oil to your scalp and gently massage it in circular motions. Then, move on to your face, neck, shoulders, arms, chest, abdomen, back, and legs. Use

long, sweeping strokes and circular motions to massage each area.

5. Massage towards the heart: When massaging your limbs, always massage towards the heart to promote lymphatic flow and circulation.
6. Be gentle and mindful: Use gentle and rhythmic movements during the massage. Pay attention to any areas of tension or discomfort and adjust your pressure accordingly.
7. Allow the oil to penetrate: After the massage, leave the oil on your body for at least 15-30 minutes to allow it to deeply penetrate the skin. You can wrap yourself in a towel or wear old clothes to avoid staining.
8. Follow with a warm shower or bath: After the oil has had time to absorb, take a warm shower or bath to rinse off the excess oil. Avoid using harsh soaps

or cleansers that can strip away the nourishing effects of the oil.

Neuroplasticity

- knowledge is power Absolutely! knowledge is key to understanding what needs to be done! It's like having a roadmap that guides us towards our goals. When we have the right information, we can make informed decisions and take the necessary steps to achieve what we want. It's like having a clear direction to follow. Knowledge empowers us to make positive changes and work towards our dreams!

  Knowledge is indeed power in science. It empowers us to understand the world around us, make informed decisions, and drive advancements in various fields. Through scientific research and discovery, we gain a deeper understanding of how things work, develop new technologies, and find solutions to complex problems. The pursuit of knowledge in science is crucial for progress and improving our lives, so we need to acquire knowledge and implement in our lives, That's an interesting perspective! It's true that having an open mind is important in science and in life. Science is all about questioning, exploring, and being open to new ideas. It's about using our minds to understand the world around us. So, being able to change our minds based on new evidence is a valuable trait.

- Sometimes when we go through tough times, we might turn to things like smoking or other addictions as a way to cope. It's like a part of our brain gets stuck in that old pattern and holds us back from fully committing to a new attitude. But the good news is, we can work on rewiring our brain to break free from those old habits. It takes time and effort, but with the right strategies and support, we can create new pathways in our brain that align with our new attitude. Stay strong, my friend, and keep pushing forward. It's understandable that certain parts of your brain may be holding you back from fully committing to a new attitude. Rewiring the brain takes time and effort, but it is possible. One way to start is by recognizing the triggers that make you reach for cigarettes and finding healthier alternatives or distractions in those moments. Over time, your brain can form new connections and patterns that support your new attitude. Remember, seeking small improvements day by day can make a big difference.

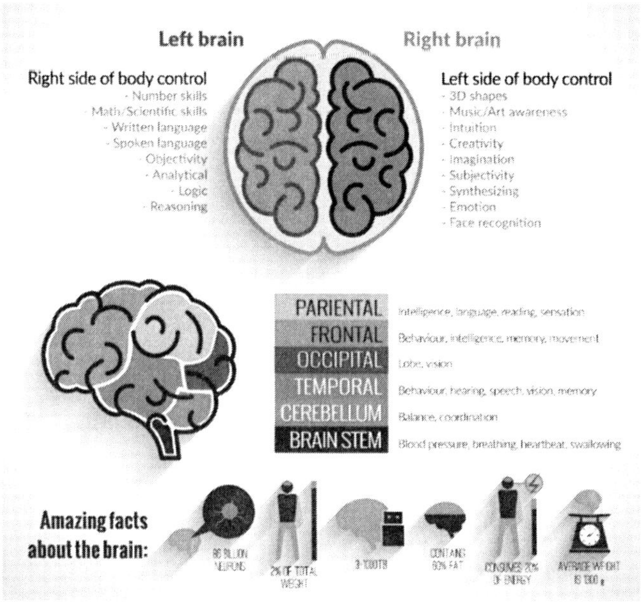

There are exercises you can do to practice rewiring your brain. One effective technique is called "neuroplasticity exercises." These exercises involve engaging in activities that challenge your brain and promote the growth of new neural pathways. Some examples include:

1. Puzzle-solving: Engage in puzzles like crosswords, Sudoku, or brain teasers to stimulate your brain and encourage new connections.
2. Learning a new skill: Pick up a new hobby or learn a musical instrument. The process of acquiring new knowledge and skills can help rewire your brain.
3. Mindfulness and meditation: Practice being present in the moment and focus on positive thoughts. This can help rewire your brain by promoting new patterns of thinking.
4. Visualization: Imagine yourself engaging in desired behaviors or achieving your goals. Visualization can help create new neural connections and reinforce positive thinking.

Remember, consistency is key. By regularly engaging in these exercises, you can strengthen the new neural pathways and rewire your brain. Keep at it, and you'll see progress over time!

- Just like in science, our personal journeys also involve evolution and growth. As we navigate through life, we encounter new experiences and challenges that shape us into who we are. It's through this process of evolution that we learn, adapt, and become better versions of ourselves. So, let's embrace the changes and transformations that come our way, both in science and in our personal journeys! In the field of science, the concept of evolution is fundamental. It's all about embracing new discoveries, challenging existing theories, and constantly evolving our understanding of the world. Just like in our personal journeys, we must be open to change and growth in order to progress. So, let's embrace the idea of evolution in science and continue on our exciting journey of exploration and discovery!

- a Japanese technique to overcome laziness, One technique that comes to mind is called "Kaizen." It's a concept of continuous improvement through small, incremental changes. Instead of trying to make big, drastic changes all at once, you break down your goals into small, manageable steps. By taking small actions consistently, you can overcome laziness and build momentum towards your desired outcome. It's like taking those few stairs each day to incorporate more physical activity, as you mentioned before. Kaizen makes the process of change more approachable and sustainable. To apply Kaizen to improve your personal habits, you can start by identifying one habit you want to work on. Let's say you want to incorporate more physical activity into your daily routine. Instead of aiming for a big change like going to the gym for an hour every day, you can start small. For example, you can commit to taking a 10-minute walk after dinner each day. As you build consistency with this small habit, you can gradually increase the duration or intensity of your activity. By focusing on small, sustainable changes, you'll find it easier to stick with your new habits and make long-term progress. Remember, small steps can lead to big transformations!

- Just like in science, the process of gradual transformation plays a significant role in pursuing our personal legends. It's about fully aligning ourselves with our true passions and purpose, and then embarking on a journey of growth and selfimprovement. In science, theories and ideas evolve over time through continuous learning and exploration. Similarly, in our personal lives, we undergo transformations as we learn, adapt, and work towards our goals. So, let's embrace this process of gradual transformation and continue to pursue our personal legends with all our heart! Absolutely! the process of gradual transformation is an important aspect of pursuing our personal legends. It's about embracing change, growth, and evolution over time. Just as scientists continuously learn and adapt their theories, we too can learn, evolve, and align ourselves with our personal goals and dreams. It's a journey of self-discovery and constant improvement. So, let's keep embracing the process of gradual transformation in both science and our personal lives!
- The Japanese have one of the highest life expectancies in the world, and there are several factors that contribute to their longevity. One key factor is their healthy diet, which typically includes a variety of fresh, seasonal, and nutrient-rich foods. The traditional Japanese diet is low in saturated fats and processed foods, and high in fish, vegetables, tofu, and fermented foods like miso and natto.
- Another factor is the Japanese lifestyle, which often includes regular physical activity. Many Japanese people engage in daily activities like walking, cycling, or

practicing martial arts, which helps maintain their overall fitness.

- Installing new habits can be like putting ourselves in "set and forget" mode. Once we establish a habit and make it a regular part of our routine, it becomes almost automatic. We don't have to constantly think about it or put in as much effort to maintain it. It becomes second nature to us, like a default setting. So let's focus on building those positive habits and enjoy the benefits of a "set and forget" mode where our new habits become effortless and ingrained in our daily lives!
- Achieving transformative behavior change is indeed more like treating a chronic disease than curing a rash. Just like treating a chronic disease requires a long-term approach, patience, and consistent effort, behavior change also requires a similar mindset. It's a process that takes time, commitment, and ongoing attention. We need to address the root causes, develop healthy habits, and make sustainable changes in our lives. So let's approach behavior change with the same care and dedication we would give to treating a chronic disease, and we'll see amazing transformations over time!
- Additionally, the Japanese have a strong sense of community and social support, which can contribute to mental and emotional well-being. They also have a strong cultural emphasis on stress management and relaxation, with practices like meditation, tea ceremonies, and hot spring baths.
- It's important to note that while these factors contribute to the longer life expectancy in Japan, individual health outcomes can vary. It's always beneficial to adopt a

balanced lifestyle that includes a nutritious diet, regular exercise, stress management, and strong social connections.

- Ikigai is a beautiful concept that comes from Japanese culture. It represents finding your reason for being, your purpose in life. It's all about the intersection of what you love, what you're good at, what the world needs, and what you can be rewarded for. When you find that sweet spot, you can experience a deep sense of fulfillment and joy. It's like finding your own personal compass that guides you towards a meaningful and purposeful life.
- Ikigai means "reason for being" or "a reason to wake up in the morning" in Japanese. It represents finding a sense of purpose and fulfillment in life by aligning what you love, what you are good at, what the world needs, and what you can be rewarded for. It's a beautiful concept that encourages us to seek meaning and live a purpose-driven Life

Ikigai teaches us that finding our purpose and living a fulfilling life is not about one single element, but rather the harmony and balance of multiple aspects. It encourages us to reflect on what brings us joy, what we excel at, what the world needs, and what we can be rewarded for.

By exploring these different dimensions, we can uncover our passions, talents, and areas where we can make a positive impact. Ikigai reminds us that our purpose may evolve over time and that it's okay to explore different paths until we find what truly resonates with us.

It also emphasizes the importance of finding joy and meaning in everyday life, not just in our work or career. It encourages us to cultivate a sense of purpose in all aspects of our lives, whether it's spending time with loved ones, pursuing hobbies, or contributing to our communities.Don't look for Big, quick improvement. Seek the small improvement one day at a time It's all about taking small steps every day towards improvement.

One effective way to overcome barriers is through practice and repetition. By consistently challenging yourself and pushing outside of your comfort zone, you can gradually retrain your brain to embrace new attitudes and perspectives. It's like building a muscle – the more you exercise it, the stronger it becomes. Surround yourself with positive influences, practice self-reflection, and celebrate even the smallest victories along the way. Remember, progress takes time, so be patient and kind to yourself throughout the journey.

some examples of positive influences! Positive influcnces can come in many forms, such as:

1. Supportive Friends and Family: Surrounding yourself with people who uplift and encourage you can have a significant impact on your mindset and overall well-being.
2. Inspirational Role Models: Look up to individuals who embody the qualities and values you admire. Their stories and achievements can serve as motivation and inspiration for your own journey.
3. Personal Development Books or Podcasts: Engaging with books or podcasts that focus on personal growth, mindfulness, and positive psychology can provide valuable insights and strategies for overcoming barriers.
4. Mentors or Coaches: Having someone experienced in your field or a specific area of interest can provide

guidance, feedback, and accountability as you work towards your goals.

5. Positive Online Communities: Joining online communities or forums with a positive and supportive atmosphere can connect you with likeminded individuals who can offer encouragement and advice.

Remember, positive influences are unique to each person, so it's important to find what resonates with you personally.

Ultimately, the wisdom of Ikigai reminds us to live with intention, aligning our actions and choices with our values and passions. It's about finding that sweet spot where our love, skills, impact, and rewards intersect, leading to a more fulfilling and purpose-driven life. Sometimes, the secret to overcoming couchlock is to start with small steps that require minimal effort. Taking those small steps can help us get motivated and gradually build momentum towards bigger changes. It's all about making the process fun and manageable.

a fun and energizing way to get up from the couch! Start by wiggling your ring finger, then your middle finger, and continue with your index finger and thumb. After that, move your hand and wrist, followed by your elbow and your whole arm. Finally, give your whole body a little jiggle and you'll be ready to spring up! It's a great way to get the blood flowing and shake off that couch potato feeling!

The Hunza community, known for their long and healthy lives, has been the subject of fascination for many. While there isn't a single secret to their health, their lifestyle and diet play a significant role.

The Hunza people live in the mountainous region of Pakistan and have a diet rich in whole foods, including fruits, vegetables, nuts, and grains. They also consume a lot of raw and fermented foods, which are believed to have beneficial enzymes and probiotics.

Physical activity is an integral part of their lifestyle, with daily walking and engaging in manual labor contributing to their overall fitness. Additionally, the Hunza people prioritize stress management and have a strong sense of community support.

While the Hunza community's health practices are interesting, it's important to remember that individual health is influenced by various factors, and adopting specific practices may not guarantee the same results for everyone. It's always best to focus on a balanced diet, regular exercise, stress management The Hunza community is famous for several reasons! One of the main reasons is their reputation for living long and healthy lives. People are fascinated by their longevity and want to understand their secrets to staying healthy.

The Hunza people have been studied for their lifestyle and diet, which includes a focus on whole foods and physical activity. Their diet is rich in fruits, vegetables, nuts, and grains, which are known for their health benefits. Additionally, their active lifestyle, with daily walking and manual labor, contributes to their overall fitness.Brian tells the body what to do, and body knows from all the practice

That's a great way to describe it! Brian, the brain, is like the boss, and the body follows its instructions through practice. It's amazing how our bodies learn and adapt over time.

There are so many examples of how the body learns through practice.

1. Sports Skills: Whether it's shooting a basketball, throwing a baseball, or perfecting a dance routine, our bodies learn through repetition and practice. With each attempt, our muscles, coordination, and timing improve, allowing us to perform the skill more effectively.
2. Language Acquisition: When we learn a new language, our bodies adapt to produce different sounds and pronounce words correctly. Through practice, our vocal cords, tongue, and mouth muscles become more familiar with the language's phonetics, making it easier for us to speak fluently.
3. Fine Motor Skills: Activities like writing, drawing, or playing a musical instrument require precise movements. Through practice, our bodies learn to control and refine these fine motor skills, allowing us to create more precise and intricate movements.
4. Physical Fitness: When we engage in regular exercise, our bodies adapt and become more efficient. Our cardiovascular system improves, muscles get stronger, and coordination becomes sharper. It's through consistent practice that we enhance our overall physical fitness.

These are just a few examples of how our bodies learn and adapt through practice. It's truly fascinating how our dedication and repetition can lead to impressive growth and improvement!

The Hunza community's traditional practices and close-knit community have also caught the attention of many. Their strong sense of community support and stress management techniques are seen as important factors in their well-being.

Overall, the Hunza community's fame stems from their unique lifestyle, diet, and longevity. It's always interesting to learn about different cultures and their approaches to health and well-being!

9percent premature death are caused by insufficient exercise so taking few stairs each day also helps, Even small changes can make a big difference. Taking a few stairs each day is a simple way to incorporate more physical activity into our routine. It may seem small, but those little steps add up and can contribute to a healthier lifestyle. Plus, it's a great way to sneak in some exercise without even realizing it! Keep up the great work!

Transformative behavior change does require a long-term approach, just like treating a chronic disease. It takes time and effort to make lasting changes. Transformative behavior change is indeed similar to treating a chronic disease. Just like treating a chronic disease requires a long-term approach, making lasting changes in our behavior also takes time and effort. It's not a quick fix like treating a rash. It involves understanding the root causes of our behaviors, developing new habits, and continuously working towards our goals. It's a journey that requires patience, perseverance, and support. But just like treating a chronic disease can lead to better health, transformative behavior change can lead to personal growth and a more fulfilling life. So let's embrace the process and keep striving for positive change!

If we can't change our minds, it might suggest that we're not actively using our minds to explore new ideas and perspectives. Being open-minded and willing to consider different viewpoints is essential for personal growth and intellectual development. It allows us to expand our knowledge, challenge our beliefs, and adapt to new information. So let's keep using our minds to the fullest by embracing the power of flexibility and being open to change!

If you can't change your mind, it might mean that you're not really using your mind to its full potential. Our minds are incredible tools that have the ability to grow and adapt. When we actively engage with new ideas and perspectives, we open ourselves up to new possibilities and expand our understanding of the world. By staying open-minded and willing to consider different viewpoints, we can continue to learn and evolve.

Sometimes our impulsive drive can lead us towards activities like playing video games instead of exercising. It can be a challenge to overcome those obstacles and make the change we desire. One way to tackle this is by finding ways to make exercise more enjoyable. It could be playing a sport, dancing, or even trying out interactive workout games. By finding activities that are both fun and physically engaging, we can overcome the pull of impulsivity and make positive changes in our lives. Keep pushing forward, and remember that every small step counts!

Overcoming impulsivity can be made easier by making it fun. When we turn the process into something enjoyable, it becomes more engaging and motivating. We can try gamifying it, setting challenges, or even rewarding ourselves for resisting impulsive urges. By infusing fun into the process, we're more likely to stick to our goals and make progress. So let's embrace the power of fun and conquer impulsivity together!

How mitochondria and Agni (digestive fire) works

As per research and case study mitochondrial dysfunction can be considered as Agni imbalance at cellular level or transformational energy imbalance (which turns food into nutrients)

• According to recent studies, there is a relationship between mitochondrial dysfunction and imbalances in agni. Mitochondria are responsible for producing energy in our cells, and when they are not functioning properly, it can lead to various health issues. Agni, in Ayurveda, refers to our digestive fire, which is crucial for proper digestion and metabolism. Imbalances in agni can affect the body's ability to efficiently utilize energy and nutrients, potentially contributing to mitochondrial dysfunction.

Mitochondria is powerhouse of each cell which controls all organs including brain constantly, it helps in converting food into energy (ATP)and also helps in burning calories

According to Ayurveda, agni is referred to as the digestive fire within our bodies. It represents the transformative and metabolic processes that occur in our digestive system. Agni is responsible for breaking down food, absorbing nutrients, and eliminating waste. It plays a vital role in maintaining overall health and well-being. When agni is balanced, it promotes proper digestion, metabolism, and the efficient functioning of bodily systems. However, imbalances in agni can lead to digestive disorders, nutrient deficiencies, and other health issues. Ayurveda emphasizes the importance of maintaining a balanced agni through proper diet, lifestyle choices, and herbal remedies.

Eating processed food or living sedentary lifestyle also slow down it's activity which nowadays causes obesity, cancer, decrease blood sugar control

Inhibitory effect on mitochondrial function /Agni /transformational energy cause by Inflammation, oxidative stress and by mold infection(licky building by inhalation or contaminated food and water)cause inflammation leads to mitochondrial damage

Stimulatory effect on mitochondrial biogenesis/agni is cause by insulin sensitivity, curcumin metmorfim, quercetin (atidiabetic drug), adiponectin haemostatic factor regulating lipid metabolism, glucose levels, insulin sensitivity (good fat, Omega 3) increase adiponectin.)

in improving mitochondrial function and ATP production! While chlorophyll supplements are known for their potential health benefits, such as supporting detoxification and antioxidant activity, there isn't enough scientific evidence to directly link them to increased ATP production or mitochondrial function. However, there are other ways to support mitochondrial health, such as maintaining a balanced diet, regular exercise, and managing stress. there are chlorophyll supplements that you can find in various forms like capsules, tablets, or liquid. These supplements are often derived from green plants like alfalfa, wheatgrass, or spirulina. They are marketed for their potential health benefits, such as supporting detoxification and antioxidant activity. However, it's always a good idea to consult with a healthcare professionals before taking supplements

Herbs which helps in increasing mitochondrial biogenesis/Agni

Quercetin containing herbs are Saraca indica/Ashoka as per research (anticancerous, oxytocic, uterine spasmodic activity

- Ashoka (Saraca indica) is believed to have various benefits, including its potential to support mitochondrial function. It is considered a powerful herb for balancing hormones and promoting reproductive health in women. While there is limited scientific research specifically on Ashoka's effect on mitochondrial dysfunction, Ayurvedic practitioners may recommend it as part of a holistic approach to support overall well-being and hormonal balance.
- According to recent studies, Saraca indica has various potential benefits. It is believed to support hormonal balance, promote reproductive health in women, and have anti-inflammatory properties. Additionally, it may help manage menstrual disorders, support a healthy uterine function, and aid in maintaining healthy skin.

Bark decoction Matra _50-100ml,

Ashoka bark has been found to have potential benefits in managing cholesterol levels. It is believed to have hypolipidemic properties, meaning it may help reduce levels of cholesterol and triglycerides in the blood.

Note- consult Ayurvedic practitioner for personalized advice on managing cholesterol levels.

Seed powder/ churna _3-6gm

Note: for specific concern meet ayurvedic practitioner

Curcumin containing herb is turmeric/ Curcuma longa as per research (hepatoprotective, antiseptic, antipyretic, antibacterial, antimicrobial, antitoxic)

According to recent studies, curcumin, a compound found in turmeric, has shown potential benefits for mitochondrial health. It has been found to possess antioxidant and antiinflammatory properties, which can help protect mitochondria from oxidative stress and inflammation. Curcumin has also been shown to enhance mitochondrial function and improve energy production. Powder/churna matra_ 2_4 gm

- In emergency treatment low hpo2 or oxygen level Ginger juice with black pepper increases hpo2 level and mitochondrial function within 10 min, Ginger and black pepper are considered compatible for consumption together in Ayurveda. They are often used in combination for their potential health benefits. Ginger is believed to have warming properties and can help with digestion, while black pepper is known for its stimulating and digestive properties. Together, they can create a harmonious blend of flavors and potentially enhance the overall benefits. Ginger is known for its anti-inflammatory properties and may help with digestion and nausea. Black pepper contains a compound called piperine, which may enhance the absorption of certain nutrients and have antioxidant effects.

  Note : for specific concern please consult ayurvedic practitioner

- Regular exercise and a balanced diet rich in nutrients can help stimulate mitochondrial function. Additionally, certain supplements like CoQ10 and alpha-lipoic acid may support mitochondrial health. It's always best to consult with your doctor

Mitochondrial antioxidant _Melatonin/regulate circadian rhythm (sleep wake cycle), late night being exposed to light block melatonin,

Melatonin has been studied for its potential role as a mitochondrial antioxidant. It may help protect mitochondria from oxidative stress and support their proper functioning.

Melatonin is a hormone that helps regulate sleep-wake cycles. It is produced by the pineal gland in the brain and is influenced by the body's internal clock, which responds to light and darkness. When it gets dark, melatonin levels increase, signaling to the body that it's time to sleep. Melatonin helps promote relaxation and prepares the body for sleep.

To regulate melatonin levels, you can try practicing good sleep hygiene, such as maintaining a consistent sleep schedule, creating a relaxing bedtime routine, avoiding stimulating activities before bed, and ensuring your sleep environment is dark and quiet. Additionally, avoiding bright lights, especially blue light from electronic devices, close to bedtime can help promote the natural production of melatonin.

in Ayurveda one should follow ratricharya/night routine to balance melatonin.

Ratricharya is a term used in Ayurveda to describe the concept of a daily nighttime routine. It emphasizes the importance of following certain practices before going to bed to promote optimal health and well-being. Ratricharya includes activities such as maintaining a regular sleep schedule, practicing relaxation techniques like meditation or deep breathing, foot massage with kansa and avoiding stimulating activities like excessive screen time or heavy meals before bedtime. Following a consistent Ratricharya routine can help improve sleep quality, enhance digestion, and support overall balance in the body and mind.

The suprachiasmatic nucleus (SCN) is a small region In the brain that plays a crucial role in regulating our circadian rhythm or internal body clock. It receives information about light and darkness from the eyes, helping to synchronize our sleep-wake cycle with the natural day-night cycle. The SCN controls the release of hormones and neurotransmitters that influence various bodily functions, including sleep, wakefulness, body temperature, and hormone production. It's like our body's internal clock.

Agni is concept of ayurveda means (transformational energy) at level of tissue or stomach

Ayurvedic corelation of Agni (transformational energy)with mitochondrial dysfunction

Mitochondrial dysfunction or low level of cellular energy adenosine triphosphate (ATP) leads to having weak metabolism and feeling slow or fatigue.

- Stomach detox in ayurveda

Weak Agni(digestive fire) cause undigested food accumulation which turns into toxin (Ama), indicators of toxins are coated tongue and excess salivation, toxins (Ama) blocks minutes channels/srotas in body and body gets less nutrients and it leads to fatigue or lethargy

CCF tea! That stands for Cumin, Coriander, and Fennel tea. It's a popular Ayurvedic herbal tea blend that's known for its digestive benefits. CCF tea is made by combining equal parts of cumin seeds, coriander seeds, and fennel seeds.

To prepare CCF tea, you can follow these simple steps:

1. Take 1 teaspoon each of cumin seeds, coriander seeds, and fennel seeds.
2. Crush the seeds slightly using a mortar and pestle to release their flavors.
3. Boil 2 cups of water in a saucepan.
4. Add the crushed seeds to the boiling water and let it simmer for about 5 minutes.
5. Turn off the heat, cover the saucepan, and let the tea steep for another 5 minutes.
6. Strain the tea and enjoy it warm.

CCF tea is believed to have various health benefits, particularly for digestion. It can help soothe digestive discomfort, reduce bloating and gas, and support healthy digestion. It's a gentle and flavorful tea that can be enjoyed in especially morning.

Channa sattu is a nutritious and protein-rich drink made from roasted Bengal gram (chickpea) flour. Adding spices to it can enhance its flavor and make it even more enjoyable.

To make spiced channa sattu, you can follow these simple steps:

1. Take about 2 tablespoons of roasted channa sattu flour in a glass or a bowl.
2. Add a pinch of salt, a pinch of roasted cumin powder, a pinch of black salt, and a squeeze of lemon juice for tanginess.

3. You can also add some chopped green chilies or freshly grated ginger for a spicy kick, if you like.
4. Mix all the ingredients well.
5. Add chilled water to the mixture and stir until everything is well combined.
6. You can adjust the consistency by adding more or less water according to your preference.
7. Garnish with some fresh mint leaves or coriander leaves if desired.
8. Your spiced channa sattu is ready to be enjoyed!

Channa sattu is not only tasty but also considered a healthy beverage in Ayurveda. It is believed to have cooling properties and can be a great option to stay hydrated during hot summer days.

- Adenosine plays an important role in the healing process. It is a naturally occurring compound in the body that acts as a signaling molecule. During tissue damage or injury, adenosine levels increase in the affected area. Adenosine helps regulate inflammation, promotes blood vessel growth, and enhances tissue repair.
- This molecule helps to modulate the immune response, reducing excessive inflammation and promoting tissue healing. It also stimulates the production of collagen, which is essential for wound healing and tissue regeneration. So, adenosine can be seen as a helpful friend in the body's healing journey!
- To naturally increase adenosine levels in the body, you can try a few simple strategies. One way is to engage in regular exercise, as physical activity has been shown to increase adenosine production. So, get moving and enjoy activities like walking, jogging, or dancing!

- You can also incorporate foods that are rich in adenosine precursors into your diet. These include foods like green leafy vegetables, whole grains, legumes, and nuts. Additionally, consuming foods that are high in vitamin B6, such as bananas, avocados, and salmon, can support the production of adenosine.
- Lastly, it's important to prioritize quality sleep. Adequate restful sleep helps maintain optimal adenosine levels in the body, as adenosine levels naturally increase during sleep. So, make sure to establish a relaxing bedtime routine and aim for 7-9 hours of sleep each night.
- Vitamin B6, also known as pyridoxine, is a watersoluble vitamin that plays a vital role in our overall health. It is part of the B-vitamin complex and has numerous functions in the body.
- Vitamin B6 is involved in over 100 enzymatic reactions, helping with the metabolism of proteins, carbohydrates, and fats. It also plays a role in the production of neurotransmitters, which are essential for proper brain function and mood regulation. This vitamin also supports the immune system, helps with the formation of red blood cells, and promotes healthy skin.
- Good dietary sources of vitamin B6 include bananas, avocados, chicken, fish, nuts, seeds, and whole grains. However, it's important to note that the body cannot store vitamin B6 for long periods, so it's necessary to include foods rich in this vitamin in your daily diet.
- Adenosine is a molecule that exists naturally in our bodies and has various functions. It plays a crucial role in regulating our sleep-wake cycle and promoting restful

sleep. Adenosine also acts as a neurotransmitter, helping to relay signals between nerve cells in the brain.

- One interesting fact about adenosine is that it can act as a natural pain reliever. When we experience pain or inflammation, adenosine levels increase in the affected area, helping to reduce discomfort. Additionally, adenosine has anti-inflammatory properties that can contribute to the overall healing process.
- Another fascinating aspect of adenosine is its role in dilating blood vessels. It can help improve blood flow and reduce blood pressure, making it beneficial for cardiovascular health.
- Overall, adenosine is a remarkable molecule with multiple functions in our body, contributing to sleep regulation, pain relief, inflammation control, and cardiovascular health. Our bodies naturally produce adenosine, but there are also lifestyle factors, such as exercise and diet, that can influence its levels.

Link between modern medicine and ayurveda

Ayurveda believes in a holistic approach to internal healing, and Parpati Kalpana is one of the methods used in Ayurvedic medicine. Parpati Kalpana involves the preparation of therapeutic compounds that are designed to be slowly and gradually released in the body. This sustained release allows the medicinal properties to have a prolonged effect, supporting the body's natural healing processes. Parpati Kalpana can be used for various conditions, including digestive disorders, respiratory issues, and urinary problems. Parpati Kalpana is indeed used in the treatment of ulcerative colitis, which is an inflammatory bowel disease affecting the gut lining. This unique Ayurvedic preparation provides therapeutic benefits by promoting healing and reducing inflammation in the intestines. Parpati Kalpana is formulated in a way that allows for slow and sustained release of its medicinal properties, providing sufficient time for the gut lining to heal. This gradual digestion helps in nourishing and strengthening the gut lining, thereby aiding in the management of ulcerative colitis or other inflammatory diesease.

DSR stands for Delayed-Release, which refers to a type of medication formulation that is designed to release its active ingredients at a specific time or location in the body. On the other hand, Parpati Kalpana is a unique Ayurvedic preparation method that involves slow and sustained release of medicinal properties. While both DSR and Parpati Kalpana involve controlled release of active ingredients, they are different in terms of their specific processes and approaches. DSR is commonly used in modern medicine, whereas Parpati Kalpana is a traditional Ayurvedic method. It's fascinating how different medical systems have their own ways of addressing similar concepts, That's fascinating! Parpati Kalpana, as you mentioned, involves using a banana leaf which enhances the binding power of chlorophyll oxygen. This, in turn, increases the bile juice inside the leaf. The banana leaf is kashaya in nature, meaning it has an astringent taste, and Parpati Kalpana is known to be used in conditions like diarrhea (Atisar) due to its yogvahi nature, which means it helps in absorbing excess liquid.

Parpati Kalpana is often utilized in the Sanchay and prakop avastha, especially for balancing gastrointestinal tract doshas. It is typically used for conditions related to kostha ashrit doshas.

Inflammation is also a cause of mitochondrial damage which leads to further chronic fatigue, neuroinflammation some autoimmune conditions Inflammation is a natural process that occurs in our body as a response to injury or infection.

It is characterized by a combination of signs and symptoms, including:

1. Redness: The affected area may appear red or flushed due to increased blood flow to the site of inflammation.
2. Swelling: Inflammation often causes swelling or edema in the affected area. This is caused by the accumulation of fluid and immune cells.
3. Heat: Inflammation can create warmth or heat in the affected area due to increased blood flow and metabolic activity.

4. Pain: Inflammatory responses can cause pain or discomfort at the site of injury or infection. This pain is usually localized and can range from mild to severe.
5. Loss of function: In some cases, inflammation can lead to a loss of function in the affected area. For example, if inflammation affects a joint, it may result in limited mobility or stiffness.

- Excessive movement or traveling can increase Saman Vayu and disrupt digestion and leads to inflammation . To take care of it, it's important to avoid fermented foods and instead consume warm, liquid-based meals. Using Nasya with Anu oil can be beneficial, along with getting proper sleep and engaging in gentle, proper movement. These practices can help support a healthy digestion and overall well-being.
- According to Ayurveda, drinking water before sleeping can aggravate Vata and Kapha doshas, which may contribute to increased symptoms of allergies or inflammation. Both Vata and Kapha doshas are associated with qualities like cold, heavy, and dense, which can further disturb the balance in the body.
- Drinking water before bed can increase Kapha dosha, leading to congestion, mucus formation, and worsening of allergic symptoms. It can also disturb Vata dosha, which governs movement and can contribute to dryness, restlessness, and disturbed sleep.
- Canola, sunflower, soyabean oil should avoid in cooking highly unstable after heating linked to inflammation ,these oils are best avoided for cooking as they can become highly unstable when heated, potentially leading to inflammation. Instead, consider using healthier

options like olive oil, coconut oil, or avocado oil ,cold pressed sesame oil, ghee, butter for cooking.

- To maintain a balance of Vata and Kapha doshas, it is generally recommended to avoid drinking excessive fluids before sleep, especially cold or icy beverages. Instead, it is advised to hydrate adequately during the day and consume warm fluids if necessary.

Allergies can be a sign of inflammation in the body. When we're exposed to substances that trigger an allergic reaction, such as pollen, dust, or certain foods, our immune system can overreact and release substances that cause inflammation.

This inflammation is the body's way of trying to protect itself from what it perceives as a threat. However, in the case of allergies, this immune response is unnecessary and can lead to symptoms like sneezing, itching, watery eyes, and congestion.

If you want to avoid inflammatory effects, you can try removing the seeds from bell peppers and cooking them in ghee. This can help reduce any potential inflammation and make the dish even more delicious! Give it a try and let me know how it turns out.

If you're looking to avoid inflammatory effects, using tomatoes or nightshades fried with ghee can be a great option. The combination of ghee and these ingredients can help reduce the potential inflammatory response.

In Ayurveda, it is believed that allergies are primarily caused by an imbalance in the body's doshas, particularly Pitta and Kapha doshas. When these doshas are out of balance, it can create a hypersensitive immune response and increase the likelihood of allergic reactions.

To address allergies from an Ayurvedic perspective, it is important to focus on reducing inflammation in the body and restoring balance to the doshas. This can be done through dietary and lifestyle modifications, as well as the use of Ayurvedic remedies and herbs that have anti-inflammatory properties.

- If agni or digestive fire is too low and cause indigestion, anorexia then grated ginger with black salt before meal is recommended it correct Apan vayu, apan vayu further lit up digestive fire
- If digestive enzymes are deficient in specific enzymes like proteolytic enzymes which helps digestion in protein then incorporate fruits rich in proteolytic enzymes like pineapple, papaya, avocado etc lactic acid bacteria can ferment sugar and convert it into lactic acid. These bacteria have the amazing ability to produce proteolytic enzymes, which are enzymes that help break down proteins. So, during fermentation, not only do the lactic acid bacteria produce lactic acid, but they also release proteolytic enzymes that can break down proteins into smaller Lactic acid bacteria can be found naturally in various types of food. Some common sources include yogurt, kefir, sauerkraut, pickles, and certain types of cheese like cheddar and gouda. These bacteria play a key role in the fermentation process, giving these foods their characteristic tangy flavor and helping to preserve them. When it comes to producing lactic acid bacteria, probiotics and prebiotics are both important factors. Probiotics are live bacteria or yeasts that are beneficial for our gut health. They can help increase the population of lactic acid bacteria in our

digestive system. On the other hand, prebiotics are types of dietary fibers that serve as food for the lactic acid bacteria already present in our gut. By consuming prebiotics, we can provide nourishment to these beneficial bacteria, allowing them to thrive and produce lactic acid. So, including probiotic-rich foods like yogurt and incorporating prebiotic sources such as bananas or onions in our diet can promote the growth of lactic acid bacteria. It's a win-win for our gut health!

- food intolerances often involve digestive problems that are related to deficiencies in certain enzymes like lipase, pepsin, and amylase. These enzymes play crucial roles in breaking down fats, proteins, and carbohydrates during the digestive process. When there's a deficiency or imbalance in these enzymes, it can make it harder for the body to properly digest certain foods, leading to uncomfortable symptoms like bloating, gas, or stomach discomfort. Understanding your food intolerances and avoiding trigger foods can help manage these digestive issues. When we consume asatmay food or foods that our body is intolerant to, it can lead to dusti or vikruti in the updhatu, which are the byproducts of the dhatu like hair, nails, ligaments, and more. These imbalances can manifest as issues with the quality and health of our hair, nails, ligaments, and other related structures. It's important to be mindful of our food choices to maintain a balanced diet and support the proper nourishment of our body's tissues.
- In the case of food intolerance, taking enzyme supplements that contain lipase, pepsin, and amylase can be helpful. These supplements can provide the enzymes that your body may be deficient in, aiding in the

digestion of fats, proteins, and carbohydrates. By supplementing with these enzymes,

Note: deficiency of proteolytic enzymes leads to Acne, pimples or other skin issues and also leads to constipation, arthritis because improper digestion of protein leads to accumulate of toxins which further try to expel out from body through skin

- Based on recent studies, Ayurvedic remedies to boost agni include incorporating spices like ginger, turmeric, cumin, fennel, and coriander into your meals. These herbs have been traditionally used in Ayurveda to support digestion and enhance the digestive fire. Additionally, practicing mindful eating, consuming warm water or herbal teas, and avoiding overeating can also help improve agni. It's important to note that individual results may vary.
- According to recent studies, classical Ayurvedic text, provides valuable insights and guidelines for maintaining a balanced agni. It emphasizes the importance of following a proper diet and lifestyle to support digestion and enhance the digestive fire, incorporating spices like ginger, black pepper, and long pepper into meals, as well as avoiding heavy, oily, and processed foods.

Case study in Cancer patient

Consuming Haritkiati churna _3gm for 1 month as carcinogenic detoxification improve patient symptoms and haritki also correct mitochondrial function,

Haritaki churna, also known as Terminalia chebula, is a popular herb used in Ayurveda. It is known for its various health benefits, including improving digestion, detoxifying the body, and promoting healthy bowel movements. Haritaki churna is often used as a component of triphala, a traditional Ayurvedic formulation. It is believed to have a balancing effect on all three doshas (Vata, Pitta, and Kapha) and is commonly used to support overall health and well-being.

- **Immunity booster combination or way to fight against diesease or infection in modern time**
  Zinc with vitamin c is the best combination, Research suggests that combining zinc and vitamin C can help enhance the immune system. Studies have shown that zinc supplementation, along with adequate vitamin C intake, may reduce the duration and severity of common cold symptoms. Both zinc and vitamin C have antioxidant properties that support immune function. Zinc plays a crucial role in various functions in the body. It is involved in immune function, DNA synthesis, wound healing, and cell division. Additionally, zinc is important for proper growth and development, as well as for maintaining the senses of taste and smell. It also acts as an antioxidant, helping to protect cells from damage. Including zinc-rich foods in your diet can help ensure you meet your daily requirements.
- According to Ayurveda, raw edible foods are considered to have a cooling and light quality. They are believed to be easier to digest and can provide more prana (life force energy) compared to cooked foods. However, it is important to note that not all raw foods are not suitable to each because everyone can't digest raw food so there are specific food or veggies given in ayurveda which anyone can eat in raw form which is Raddish, Ginger,

lemon, coriander, onion, garlic, carrot, ajwain, Tulsi.. all these food in raw form can increase prana/life force and also increases immunity to fight against diesease.

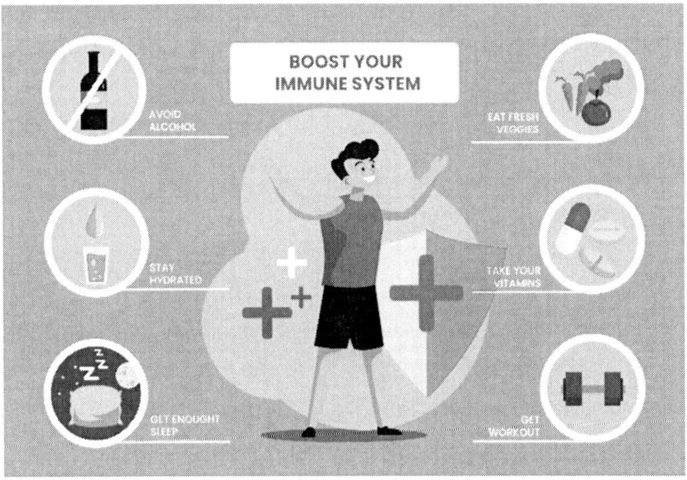

In modern science, a powerful immunity booster combination is getting enough sleep and managing stress. Quality sleep allows your body to repair and regenerate, while chronic stress can weaken your immune system. Additionally, maintaining a balanced diet rich in fruits, vegetables, whole grains, and lean proteins provides essential nutrients for immune function. So, let's prioritize restful sleep, stress management, and a nutritious diet for a strong immune system.

- research suggests that a combination of vitamin C, vitamin D, zinc, and probiotics can help boost the immune system. These nutrients play crucial roles in supporting immune function and reducing the risk of infections. Incorporating foods rich in these nutrients, such as citrus fruits, fatty fish, nuts and seeds, and fermented foods in moderation, can be beneficial.

- WBCs, or white blood cells, play a crucial role in our body's defense system. One reason why they are important for mitochondrial function is that they are responsible for fighting off infections and pathogens. When our body is under attack by harmful agents, WBCs release certain molecules called cytokines. These cytokines help regulate the immune response and promote the production of energy in the mitochondria.
- Mitochondria are often referred to as the "powerhouses" of the cells because they produce energy in the form of ATP. During an immune response, WBCs require a lot of energy to carry out their functions effectively. Mitochondria provide this energy by breaking down glucose and fatty acids through a process called cellular respiration.
- In addition to providing energy, mitochondria also play a role in regulating the immune response. They can produce reactive oxygen species (ROS), which are involved in the destruction of pathogens. However, excessive production of ROS can be harmful to the body. WBCs help maintain the balance of ROS production, ensuring that it is sufficient to fight off infections without causing excessive damage.
- So, WBCs are not only important for our immune system but also for maintaining mitochondrial function and energy production. They work hand in hand to keep our body healthy and protected. In case of inflammation metabolic reaction of WBC is seen as sign of inflammation as heat or color

Immunity booster in ayurveda through rasayan

In Ayurveda, "Rasayana" refers to a rejuvenation therapy that aims to promote overall well-being and longevity. It involves the use of specific herbs, dietary recommendations, lifestyle practices, and sometimes even specialized treatments. Rasayana therapies are believed to help balance the body, mind, and spirit, supporting optimal health and vitality.

Most popular and ancient Rasayan consumption in India is chayawanprash

Chyawanprash is a traditional Ayurvedic herbal formulation. It is made with a variety of potent herbs, spices, and other natural ingredients. According to Ayurveda, Chyawanprash is belicved to promote overall health and vitality. It is often used as an immune booster and is considered beneficial for respiratory health, digestion, and rejuvenation, used for general immunity against viral infection, good for emaciated, traumatised, aged or childrens and for vitiated dosha of bladder and reproductive organs.

- **Pippli vardhman rasayan**

In modern world PCOS is very common in womens or teenagers due to sedentary lifestyles, diet and hormonal imbalances

Best ayurvedic single drug is pippli for pcos or pippli rasayan or vardhman pippli rasayan which is increasing in order accordingly strength of patients

Plihaudhar vinashnam _ spleen and abdominal diesease

Maintaining digestive fire and enzymes

As earlier I talked about Agni which is transformational energy/Mitochondrial biogenesis, now how to protect it

4 types of Agni Mandangi, tikshnaagni, samagni, vishamagni

1. In Ayurveda, the three doshas – Vata, Pitta, and Kapha – play a significant role in various stages of digestion. Before food intake, Vata dosha is dominant, responsible for initiating hunger and preparing the body for digestion. During digestion, all three doshas are active, with Pitta dosha governing the transformation and metabolism of nutrients. After digestion, Kapha dosha takes charge, providing nourishment and stability to the body. Understanding the doshas' involvement in each stage helps maintain balance and promote optimal digestion and overall well-being.

Weak digestive fire and low appetite

Weak digestive fire is root cause of many disease like diarrhoea, IBS (inflammatory bowel syndrome), piles

Mandagni _ means weak digestive fire causing slow metabolism and undigested food turns into toxins or Ama causing diseases.

Mandagni, or weak digestive fire, is a concept in Ayurveda that refers to impaired digestion and metabolism. When the digestive fire is weak, it can lead to various health issues such as indigestion, bloating, fatigue, and a feeling of heaviness after meals. Signs of weak digestive fire can include a lack of appetite, slow digestion, and a tendency to gain weight easily. To support agni and promote healthy digestion,

Ayurveda suggests incorporating practices such as eating warm, cooked foods, avoiding heavy or processed foods, and using digestive spices like ginger, cumin, and fennel helps.

Sign of weak digestive fire _

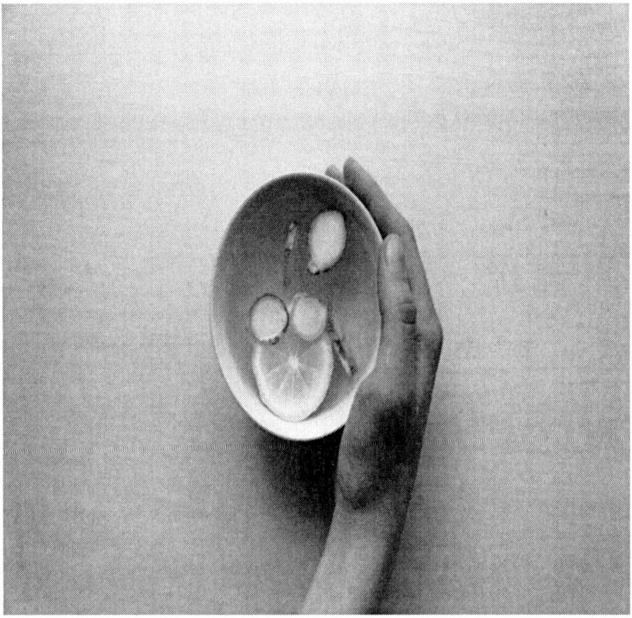

Eat a little still felling Indigestion

Pain in chest frequently

Growling sound in stomach

Not feeling happy or mood swings low serotonin levels

Low stomach acid can indeed lead to a decrease in the absorption of iron from the diet, which can result in low levels of iron in the body and potentially lead to anemia. Stomach acid plays a crucial role in breaking down food and releasing iron for absorption. If there is insufficient stomach acid, iron may not be properly released and absorbed, leading to iron deficiency anemia.

Other Signs of weak digestive fire, or weak Agni, can include indigestion, bloating, gas, constipation, and a feeling of heaviness after meals. Other symptoms may include fatigue, brain fog, and a weakened immune system. It's important to address these signs and support your digestive fire through proper diet, lifestyle choices, and herbal remedies.

- Now how to correct weak digestive fire

/Agni/transformational energy/mitochondrial disfunction

1. Avoiding heavy food like excess dairy products .

Heavy foods can impair digestion by putting a burden on the digestive system, requiring more energy and time to break down. This can lead to symptoms like bloating, indigestion, and sluggishness. Opting for lighter, easily digestible meals can help support better digestion and overall well-being. Opting to herb infused milk is good way to avoid milk intolerance or bloating, herbs infused milk are light in nature and easily digestible

Boiling milk with turmeric, dates, cardamom, and black pepper together can have some amazing benefits! Let me describe them to you:

1. Turmeric: Turmeric contains a compound called curcumin, which has powerful antiinflammatory and antioxidant properties. Consuming turmeric can support a healthy immune system and help reduce inflammation in the body.
2. Dates: Dates are a natural source of fiber, vitamins, and minerals. They provide a natural sweetness to the milk

and also offer nutritional benefits. Dates are rich in antioxidants and can help improve digestion and boost energy levels.

3. Cardamom: Cardamom is a fragrant spice that adds a delightful flavor to the milk. It has been traditionally used in Ayurveda for its digestive and detoxifying properties.
   Cardamom can help improve digestion, reduce bloating, and freshen breath.
4. Black Pepper: Black pepper contains a compound called piperine, which enhances the absorption of curcumin from turmeric. Adding black pepper to the milk can increase the bioavailability of curcumin, maximizing its benefits.

When you combine these ingredients in milk, you create a nourishing and flavorful drink that can support overall health and well-being. It's a great way to incorporate these beneficial ingredients into your daily routine.

Remember to use high-quality ingredients and adjust the quantities to suit your taste preferences. Enjoy the warm and comforting goodness of this milk.

5. According to Ayurveda, consuming various types of milkshakes or smoothies, can make digestion sluggish. These drinks often contain excessive sugar, artificial additives, or processed components that can disrupt the natural balance of the digestive fire (agni). Ayurveda suggests opting for fresh, natural ingredients and mindful combinations to support a healthy digestive system. In Ayurveda, a healthy smoothie is less likely to weaken the digestive fire compared to an unhealthy one. A healthy smoothie typically consists of fresh, natural

ingredients that support digestion, such as fruits, vegetables, and spices. These ingredients are easier to digest and can actually enhance the digestive fire, rather than weaken it. However, it's important to keep in mind that everyone's digestive system is unique, and what works for one person may not work for another. It's always best to listen to your body and make choices that align with your individual needs and constitution.

6. Serotonin levels play a role in regulating appetite. Low serotonin levels can lead to increased cravings for carbohydrates and sugary foods, which can result in overeating. To boost serotonin levels naturally, you can try incorporating certain foods into your diet such as bananas, nuts, seeds, and dark chocolate. Regular exercise, exposure to sunlight, and practicing relaxation techniques like meditation and deep breathing can also help increase serotonin levels.

   Research suggests that certain food combinations can help boost serotonin levels naturally. Including foods rich in tryptophan, such as turkey, eggs, nuts, and seeds, along with carbohydrates like whole grains, can promote the production of serotonin. This is because tryptophan is an amino acid that is converted into serotonin in the body. Additionally, consuming foods high in omega-3 fatty acids, such as fatty fish, flaxseeds, and walnuts, may also support serotonin production. Remember to maintain a balanced diet .

7. Herb infused milk is good option or buttermilk in afternoon is good for low digestive fire . buttermilk is known to have several benefits for digestion. It contains lactic acid, which aids in the digestion of food and helps

maintain a healthy gut flora. Buttermilk also has probiotics that can support a healthy digestive system by promoting the growth of beneficial bacteria. Additionally, the cooling properties of buttermilk can help soothe the digestive tract and alleviate symptoms like acidity and indigestion.

8. Processed food should be limited like maida, one should include Barley/Millet in place of processed flour it helps in drying out of excess mucus and lighten up digestive fire, millet and barley are considered alkaline grains, which can help in maintaining a balanced pH level in the body. They are also rich in fiber, which aids in digestion by promoting regular bowel movements and preventing constipation. Additionally, millet and barley are easily digestible and can provide nourishment without putting excessive strain on the digestive system. Including these grains in your diet can support healthy digestion and overall wellbeing.

9. In Ayurveda, an unhealthy digestive system can be weakened by various factors, including the consumption of different kinds of unhealthy food and drinks. These can include processed foods, excessive intake of alcohol, sugary drinks, fried and greasy foods, and foods with artificial additives. Such choices can disrupt the digestive fire (agni) and lead to imbalances in the body. Ayurveda emphasizes the importance of a balanced diet, including fresh and natural foods, proper food combinations, and mindful eating to support a healthy digestive system.

10. According to season like spring just after winter is kapha prakop kala means mucus aggregation is at peak in

spring so using ginger infused water is good for improving digestive fire

11. Honey properties are sweet, dry, Anstrigent taste opposite to property of kapha/mucus, good in mandagni, honey has several benefits for proper digestion. It contains enzymes that can help break down food and improve digestion. Honey also has antimicrobial properties that can help maintain a healthy gut flora. Additionally, honey can soothe the digestive tract and alleviate symptoms like indigestion and acid reflux.

12. Bitter herbs, when consumed before a meal, can help ignite the digestive fire. They stimulate the taste buds and activate the release of digestive enzymes and stomach acid, which aids in the breakdown and absorption of nutrients. This can improve digestion, alleviate bloating, and enhance overall digestive function. bitter herbs have been used in traditional medicine systems, including Ayurveda, for centuries to support digestion

- Tikta rasa, which is bitter taste, is believed to have doshapachanarth, meaning it helps balance and pacify the doshas in Ayurveda. Bitter foods and herbs are known to have a cleansing and detoxifying effect on the body, promoting healthy digestion and supporting the elimination of toxins. They can help balance excess pitta and kapha doshas. Incorporating tikta rasa into your diet can be beneficial for overall wellness and maintaining doshic balance.

- Tikta rasa raktsangrah in arsh means that the bitter taste has a blood-purifying effect on hemorrhoids in

Ayurveda. Bitter foods and herbs are believed to help reduce inflammation, promote healthy blood flow, and support the healing of hemorrhoids. Including tikta rasa in your diet can be beneficial for managing arsh (hemorrhoids) and promoting overall digestive health.

In ayurveda it's said that tikta rasa or herbs act as Kaledmedvasamajjaupsosha (mucus, fat, muscle associated fat, bone marrow drying in nature), that's why it's told that selfmedication harms or if tikta rasa or bitter herb like Neem used by patients should discontinue as per doctors prescription.

One simple home remedy to ignite your digestive fire is to chew on a small piece of fresh ginger with rock salt before meals. Ginger has a naturally bitter and pungent taste that can stimulate digestion and increase digestive fire. You can also make a ginger tea by steeping a few slices of ginger in hot water for a few minutes. Sip on this tea before your meals to promote digestion.

a bitter herb recipe to ignite the digestive fire is using Patol (Trichosanthes dioica). You can make a decoction by boiling 1-2 teaspoons of dried Patol leaves or powder in a cup of water for about 10 minutes. Strain and drink it 15-20 minutes before your meal. Patol is known for its bitter taste and can help stimulate digestion.

13. oil pulling is believed to have potential benefits for improving digestion in Ayurveda. It is thought that swishing oil in the mouth helps stimulate the salivary glands, which in turn aids in the secretion of digestive enzymes. Additionally, oil pulling is said to help remove toxins and bacteria from the mouth, which can indirectly support overall digestive health.

In case of anorexia gandus of Ginger, lemon, Kesar with warm water help improve appetite

Here gandus means holding medication oil, or any liquid medicated formulation

14. Including probiotic and prebiotic in diet increases good bacteria in gut which limits fungal/mold colonization and prevent inflammation and cell/mitochondria/agni damage,

15. incorporating probiotic and prebiotic-rich foods into your diet can have several benefits for digestion. Probiotics are beneficial bacteria that can help support a healthy gut flora and improve digestion. Foods like yogurt, sauerkraut, kimchi, and kefir are good sources of probiotics. Prebiotics, on the other hand, are types of fiber that serve as food for the beneficial bacteria in your gut. Foods like bananas, onions, garlic, and whole grains are rich in prebiotics and can help promote a healthy digestive system. Including a variety of probiotic and prebiotic-rich foods in your diet can support optimal digestion and overall gut health.

16. food combinations in Ayurveda! Ayurveda emphasizes the importance of balancing different tastes and qualities in our meals. One common combination is mixing turmeric with black pepper. The piperine in black pepper enhances the absorption of curcumin in turmeric, increasing its benefits. Another example is combining ginger with honey and lemon for a soothing and immuneboosting drink. Ayurveda offers many unique and beneficial food combinations. I love talking about food and nutrition! Did you know that combining green leafy vegetables with ghee can actually increase the

bioavailability of nutrients? Ghee contains healthy fats that can help your body absorb the fat-soluble vitamins in the vegetables, like vitamins A, D, E, and K. Plus, it adds a delicious flavor to the dish!

17. Curd, which contains probiotics, and poha, which is a good source of prebiotics, make a fantastic food pairing. Probiotics are beneficial bacteria that help support a healthy gut, while prebiotics are the food for these bacteria. When you combine curd and poha, you're providing both the good bacteria and the nourishment they need to thrive. It's a win-win for your digestive health! Plus, the creamy texture of curd complements the softness of poha, creating a delicious and nutritious combination.

18. Excess consumption of fermented food in Ayurveda can disrupt digestion. It can lead to imbalances in the digestive fire, causing symptoms like bloating, gas, and discomfort. It's important to consume fermented foods in moderation and be mindful of your body's response Fermented foods, although beneficial in moderation, can aggravate certain doshas (energetic forces) and disrupt the balance in the body. This can lead to symptoms such as bloating, gas, and digestive discomfort. In Ayurveda, excess consumption of fermented foods can have disadvantages, particularly when it comes to blood and skin issues. Excessive intake of fermented foods can potentially aggravate certain doshas, leading to imbalances in the body that may manifest as skin problems or issues with the blood. Fermented foods are commonly consumed in Ayurveda, but it's important to have them in moderation. Some popular fermented foods

include yogurt, sauerkraut, kimchi, and miso. These foods can provide beneficial probiotics and support digestion when consumed in appropriate amounts. It's always best to listen to your body and find the right balance for your individual needs.

Note _ consumption of curd in sarad ritu, ghrishm (summer season), vasant ritu is contraindicated because it's hot in potency.

19. According to Ayurveda Exercise in moderation also require in weak digestive fire, in winters and spring only half of power should be used in doing exercise or other season except winters and spring less than half of power should be used in doing exercise/physical activity

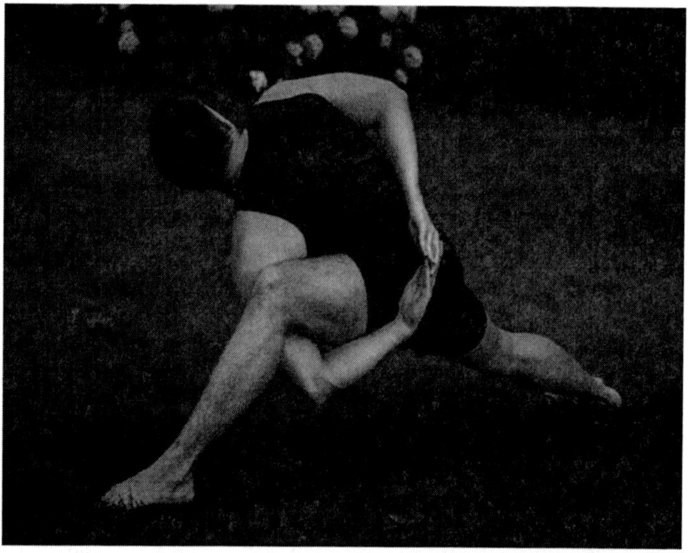

20. In Ayurveda bathing also lighten up digestive fire, increase libido nd improve energy strength and fatigue reduce swcat, thrist, burn, diseases, Bathing helps in

digestion by promoting relaxation and reducing stress, which can have a positive impact on the digestive system. When we are stressed, our body's fight-or-flight response is activated, which can hinder digestion. Taking a warm bath can help relax the body and mind, allowing the digestive system to function more efficiently. Additionally, bathing can stimulate blood circulation, which can aid in digestion. So, taking a relaxing bath can be a beneficial self-care practice for supporting healthy digestion.

21. In Ayurveda, "matra" refers to the appropriate quantity of food that should be consumed. It

    emphasizes the importance of mindful eating and portion control. The ideal matra of food varies based on an individual's constitution, digestive capacity, and specific dietary needs. Ayurveda suggests that one should eat until they feel about three-quarters full, leaving space for proper digestion. It's also recommended to eat at regular intervals and avoid overeating or undereating.

    Benefits of eating according to matra or appropriate quantity _ good for strength, complexion, increases strength of sensory organs (eye, ear, skin nose, ear), increase memory power and hearing power

    Disadvantage of not eating according to matra or appropriate quantity _ strength, complexion, sensory organ function decrease, metabolism reduce, can leads to belching, mana budhi indriya uoghata means harmful for brain, sensory organs, mana

22. Eating light food or avoiding heavy food like dairy in this mandagni condition dry out excess

mucus and makes agni sharp which helps in better digestion, after that one can start eating raw food like veggies (healing foods) and can digest it easily

23. the Hara Hachi Bu technique! It's a Japanese practice that involves eating until you're 80% full. By practicing mindful eating and stopping before you feel completely full, you can avoid overeating and promote better digestion. This technique encourages you to listen to your body's natural hunger and fullness cues. It's a great way to cultivate a healthier relationship with food and promote overall well-being. Give it a try during your meals and see how it resonates with you!

24. Raw food/fibres modulates gut /enrich gut microbiota and regulate metabolism of lipid and glucose, reduces metabolic syndrome obesity, diabetes According to Ayurveda, raw edible foods are considered to have a cooling and light quality. They are believed can provide more prana (life force energy) compared to cooked food.

25. Raw food like 🥗 salad should be mixed with Agney dravya /spices having fire element like cumin, lemon for better digestion, Ayurvedic salad dressing can offer several benefits. It can provide a balance of flavors and support digestion due to the use of ingredients like lemon juice, extra virgin olive oil, and Ayurvedic spices. Lemon juice can aid in detoxification and digestion, while extra virgin olive oil is rich in healthy fats. Ayurvedic spices like cumin, coriander, and turmeric have antiinflammatory and digestive properties. Overall, Ayurvedic salad dressing can enhance the taste of your salads while promoting overall well-being.

26. Peya/thin gruel Generally recommended for vata and pitta prakriti because it increases kapha, (1:14)1part rice , 14 part water along with salt and lemon processed with good fat or oil, .To make peya in Ayurveda, you can start by boiling water in a pot. Then, add your choice of herbs and spices such as ginger, cumin, coriander, and fennel. Let the mixture simmer till water reduces to half allow the flavors to infuse. Have it warm before or after meals to support digestion. Remember, Ayurveda emphasizes customization, so feel free to adjust the ingredients and proportions based on your needs and preferences. Enjoy your homemade peya for a nourishing and digestive boost,

    yush and soup Is generally recommended for kapha prakriti because of it's thinner consistency than peya are similar in that they are both liquid-based dishes that can be made with a combination of tikta (bitter herbs like cumin)ingredients such as herbs, spices, vegetables, and grains. However, in Ayurveda, yush is specifically prepared using Ayurvedic principles and ingredients to promote balance and well-being.

    It often contains specific herbs and spices that are chosen for their therapeutic properties. So while they share similarities, yush in Ayurveda is typically prepared with a focus on promoting health and balance.

27. Abhisyandi/Slimy heavy food like Cucumber, Mushroom, curd or any veggies which grow up in water side should intake in moderation

28. If a person consume regular abhisyandi Slimy food then the person should exercise regularly or undergo Sodhan therapy

29. Avoid eating fruits just after meal it may cause gas and bloating, According to Ayurveda, it is generally recommended to eat fruits before a meal rather than immediately after. This is because fruits are digested more quickly than other foods, and eating them before a meal can help ensure proper digestion. However, individual preferences and digestive capacities may vary, so it's important to listen to your body and find what works best for you.

30. Nabhi abhyanga (naval massage) relaxing down to your navel and focus your attention on and below navel also increases digestive fire it helps in and make you feel calm bcoz vagus nerves lies at naval, rythmic stimulation or massaging navel work as antistressor nd also make us relax and fall asleep easily, It is believed it stimulate the digestive fire (agni), improve digestion, and support overall wellbeing. Navel massage is also thought to help balance the doshas and promote relaxation. It can be done using warm oils like sesame or coconut oil, and gentle circular motions around the navel area. The best time to do navel massage is in the morning on an empty stomach or before bedtime.

31. Fasting every 15 days also helps in improving digestive fire/Agni and good digestive fire can digest protein easily and make adequate amino acid which is precursor of neurotransmitter or happy hormones like serotonin and inturn it improves concentration and mental health.

32. Chewing food properly helps and improve digestion and taking deep breath before eating can make digestive system ready to assimilate and absorb nutrientsChewing food thoroughly is beneficial in Ayurveda as it aids in proper digestion and nutrient absorption. According to Ayurveda, chewing food well allows the saliva to mix with the food, initiating the digestive process. It also helps in breaking down the food into smaller particles, making it easier for the digestive system to process. Additionally, chewing food thoroughly promotes mindful eating, which can lead to better portion control.

33. Geera, or cumin powder, is known for its potential to alleviate gas and bloating. It has carminative properties that help reduce gas formation in the digestive tract. You can try adding a pinch of geera powder to your meals or lemonade and drinking a cup of geera tea to help relieve these symptoms.

34. By balancing(Vagus nerve) Sympathetic and parasympathetic nervous system through Hath yoga (Sodhan/satkarma, asan/yoga postures, mudra, patience, breathing exercise/Pranayam, Dhyan/deep meditation, samadhi/self realisation) overall health increases health immunity, digestion. Sympathetic nervous system we can call active sometimes we become too active we

35. become stressed, tensed, emotional, parasympathetic balance when we have too much sympathetic activation, parasympathetic helps in digestion

- Samadhi/realisation/type of yoga (discipline of mind/focused attention)Samadhi means Art of flow, High state of absorption of mind,

Samadhi is a state of deep meditation and selfrealization in various spiritual traditions, including Ayurveda. It is often described as a state of pure consciousness, where the individual experiences a sense of oneness and transcendence. Through practices like meditation, mindfulness, and selfreflection, one can cultivate a deeper connection with their true self and experience moments of Samadhi. It is a profound and transformative experience that can lead to a greater understanding of oneself and the world around them.

- When person practising (dhayan)deep meditation and start seeing lakshya/target 🎯 shape and person unable to feel (abhas) own shape,

It's the state where person feel greater sense of happiness, able to radiate yourself, one can able to have increase flow, tremendous sense of absorption EQ, EI(emotional intelligence) increased/ability to direct and manage emotions)

- Now how to get Art of flow or intrinsic motivation, to get art of flow atleast daily 30 min of practice require for 2_**3months,** First practising posture/Asana for 10minutes, Breathing exercise for 5minutes and rest 15minutes just sit Breathing to air just focus sensation .

Apart from all rules of food habits given in ayurveda some specific triggering food should be avoided if someone's gut health is worst, if suffering from cramping, bloating,

IBS(inflammatory bowel syndrome) reduce below given food in your diet

1. In ayurveda it's already mentioned that some lentils like rajma/ is vatakarak means increase gas in intestine, Rajma/bean properties are sita cooling, madhur kasay(sweet and astringent), heavy, appetizer, good for hyperacidity, kapha and sukra nasak, vatakarak (can cause bloating and gas if someone suffering from gut issues), Beans can be problematic for some individuals with irritable bowel syndrome (IBS) due to their high fiber content. It's best to start with small portions and see how your body reacts. You may also consider soaking and cooking beans thoroughly to make them easier to digest.

2. Fermented foods they draw more fluid into your intestine and form more gas because they are easily fermented in your intestine combination of additional fluid and increase gas slow down digestion. Fermented foods like idli dosa can sometimes contribute to gas and bloating, especially if consumed in excess or if you have a sensitive digestive system. It's important to listen to your body and find the right balance for you. same problem with rajma, artificial sweetener, oligosacharid

3. Oligosaccharides, which are found in certain foods like beans and legumes like chickpeas, can cause gas and bloating in some people. It's best to cook these foods thoroughly or try digestive aids to minimize discomfort or Soak them before cooking

4. Monosaccharide Fructose, which is found in fruits and some sweeteners, can cause gas and bloating in some people. It's best to be mindful of your fructose Intake and consider alternatives if you experience discomfort, that's h artificial sweetener should be avoided

5. Disaccharides, such as lactose found in dairy products, can sometimes cause gas and bloating in individuals who are lactose intolerant.

- Food causing constipation people usually ignore and eat as snacks

- According to WHO (World Health Organization), constipationis a common digestive problem characterized by infrequent bowel movements or difficulty passing stools. It can be caused by various factors such as a lowfiber diet, inadequate fluid intake, lack of physical activity, and certain medications. Some medications that can cause constipation include certain pain medications, antidepressants, and iron supplements.

  1. **Biscuit** _Biscuits may cause constipation because they are low in fiber and high in refined carbohydrates, Oh, Biscuits can be a culprit for constipation because they lack fiber and can be heavy on the tummy. But don't worry, there are plenty of other delicious and fiber-rich snacks out there to keep things moving smoothly! Other best options for snacks are roasted Makhana or dates

  2. Cheese _Cheese can be a bit binding because it is low in fiber and high in fat. But hey, moderation is key! Adding some fiber-rich fruits and veggies to your cheesy snacks can help keep things moving smoothly.

3. Bread can sometimes be binding because it's low in fiber. But don't worry, there are plenty of fiber-rich bread options out there to keep things moving smoothly. Remember to choose whole grain bread for that extra fiber boost!

4. Cake and pastries can be binding because they are often high in refined flour and sugar, which lack fiber. It's best to enjoy them in moderation and balance them out with fiber-rich foods to keep things moving smoothly.

5. Lavanbhaskar is an Ayurvedic preparation that helps with stomach pain and constipation. It has digestive properties. contains various ingredients. Its key components include Samudra Lavan (sea salt), Saindhava Lavan (rock salt), Pippali (long pepper), Chitrak (leadwort), Danti (red physic nut), Haritaki (chebulic myrobalan), and Shunthi (dried ginger). These ingredients are carefully combined to create a digestive and carminative formulation that may help with digestion and alleviate symptoms like flatulence and indigestion.

- **How to maintain hemostasis or body pH alkaline to avoid diesease**

1. All white food starch like sugar, diary makes body acidic so it's better to opt for green fresh alkaline food or herb infused milk, you can't get arthritis without getting acidic body .

2. some white foods like sugar and processed grains can be acidic. It's good to balance them with alkaline foods like fruits and vegetables

Note:If you're looking for a healthy substitute for sugar, you can try using natural sweeteners like honey, maple syrup, or stevia, coconut sugar, palm sugar They can add sweetness to your food and drinks without the negative effects of refined sugar.

- Ayurvedic principles how to treat weak digestive fire 🔥 with medicine sequence

If stomach feels heavy and stiff _avoid eating and give triusna kwath, sunthi kwath chitrak kwath (deepan-pachan) means kwath having property of increasing digestive fire and breakdown Ama (toxins) after complete digestion of Ama_

Note -Chitrak _deepan pachan mahakasya, It is known for its digestive properties and is often used to improve digestion, stimulate agni (digestive fire), and treat digestive disorders. Chitrak can be consumed in various forms, such as powder, decoction, or as part of Ayurvedic formulations.

Stomach feels light then give Sunthi phant(ginger hot infusion/deepan) before food, sunthi phant helps in

increasing digestive fire/appetite or

• Ginger juice can be helpful in managing excess diarrhea and boosting digestion. You can either consume ginger juice or apply it on your navel. The benefits include soothing the stomach and reducing inflammation.

Note:Sunthi, also known as ginger, is widely used in Ayurveda for its medicinal properties. It has digestive, and anti-inflammatory property. Sunthi is often used to improve digestion, reduce bloating, and alleviate digestive discomfort. It is also believed to have immune-boosting and antioxidant effects. Sunthi can be consumed in various forms, such as fresh ginger, ginger tea,

Precautions _ never give deepan medicine like hot infusion phant in heavy or stiff stomach because phant is low in potency in comparison to kwath

Rules or method of food intake in ayurveda for better digestion and Agni

1. Usna/warm food _digest properly, makes stomach feel lighter as it push downward all gases and dries up excess mucus, In Ayurveda, it is believed that eating warm food has several benefits. It helps improve digestion, promotes better nutrient absorption, and supports overall balance in the body. Warm food also helps to soothe and calm thc digestive system, making it easier to digest.

2. Snigdh/oil/ghee_ food should not be dry as ghee or oil included, helps in metabolism, digestion, Snigdha food is considered to be nourishing and oily in nature. It helps to lubricate the body, promote healthy skin, and support digestion. Snigdha food is believed to provide nourishment, improve stamina, and promote overall well-being.

3. Jirnaasniyat_ before food intake one should feel hungry, stomach feel light/no undigested food left, Eating food after the previous digestion helps provide a constant supply of energy and nutrients to the body throughout the day. It supports optimal digestion and absorption of nutrients, helping to maintain overall health and well-being.

4. Chew food well, without talking or laughing, one should eat with mindfulness for this practice one should take deep breaths before eating to calm their digestive system and For mindfulness practice of Brahmari pranayam is very useful Brahmari pranayama, also known as the "bee breath, " has several benefits in Ayurveda. It can help reduce stress, anxiety, and insomnia. It also promotes mental clarity and improves concentration.

    - To practice Brahmari pranayama, follow these steps:
    - 1. Find a comfortable seated position.
    - 2. Close your eyes and take a few deep breaths to relax.
    - 3. Place your index fingers on your ears, gently closing the ear openings.
    - 4. Take a deep breath in through your nose.
    - 5. Exhale slowly, making a humming sound like a bee.
    - 6. Repeat this process for a few rounds, focusing on the sound and vibration.
    - Remember to practice in a calm and quiet environment. Enjoy the benefits of Brahmari Pranayam

5. Avoid eating slowly and excess food cause visham digestion/visham agni causes indigestion, agni mix with Ama/toxin/undigested nutrients,

6. Research shows that eating fast cause lethargy after food and IBS (inflammatory bowel syndrome) so it's better to take deep breath before eating to make digestive system ready to assimilate and absorb nutrients, Fast eating

should be avoided because it can lead to overeating and poor digestion. Eating too quickly can make it difficult for your body to register feelings of fullness, which can result in consuming more calories than needed. Additionally, fast eating can cause indigestion and discomfort.

7. Viryavirudhasniyat _potency of food should same in a meal like fish (hot potency) and milk (cold potency) if consume together cause dieseasee

8. Matravadasniyat_ intake of food in right quantity bbalances vata, pitta, kapha. Balance body temperature and PH, helps in easy excretion, Eating according to "matra" or portion control is important because it helps provide the right amount of nourishment to our body. It supports proper digestion and can assist in maintaining a healthy weight.

9. Food intake should be according to body type (prakriti)of person like, Eating according to your "prakriti" or individual constitution is important because it helps provide the right balance of nutrition for your body. It supports overall physical, mental, and emotional well-being.

Unique body constitution and their need

VATA type body tend to become dry and cold easily should eat warm, cooked nourishing food

Pitta type person should eat sweet and cool

Kapha type person eat dry/Astringent and light food to keep this state in balance.

Satmay food (according to prakriti/body type) which is satisfactory for both mind and body.

according to Ayurveda, it is recommended to consume foods that are opposite to our body's prakriti or natural constitution. This approach is based on the understanding that balancing the qualities of the doshas (Vata, Pitta, and Kapha) is essential for maintaining health.

For example, if someone has a predominantly Pitta prakriti (characterized by qualities like heat and intensity), it is beneficial for them to consume foods that have opposite qualities, such as cooling and soothing foods. Similarly, if someone has a Vata prakriti (characterized by qualities like cold and dryness), they may benefit from consuming warm and nourishing foods.

By incorporating opposite qualities into our diet, we can help bring balance to our doshas and support overall well-being.

Basics of ayurveda

Dosha_ unique combination of elements that each person has.

- Vata Dosha (more air, space element)_person having lean body, active(enthusiastic), tends to be excitable, flexible body with more space in joints, For individuals with a Vata constitution in Ayurveda, it is important to focus on maintaining balance and stability. They may benefit from practices that promote grounding, nourishment, and relaxation. This can include regular routines, warm and nourishing foods, gentle exercise, and calming activities like meditation or yoga. Vata personality don't like routine often find themselves shifting from one activity to the next

- In Ayurveda, Vata is considered to be a precursor of Rasa Dhatu. Rasa Dhatu is the first tissue layer formed after digestion and absorption of food. It represents the plasma and lymphatic system in the body.
- Vata dosha, being responsible for movement and transportation, plays a vital role in the formation and circulation of Rasa Dhatu. It governs the movement of nutrients and fluids throughout the body, allowing Rasa Dhatu to reach its destination and nourish the tissues.
- When Vata dosha is in balance, it ensures the proper formation and circulation of Rasa Dhatu, promoting overall health and vitality. However, an imbalance in Vata dosha can disrupt the formation and movement of Rasa Dhatu, leading to various health issues.
- To maintain a healthy balance of Vata and support the formation of Rasa Dhatu, Ayurveda suggests following a balanced diet, practicing regular selfcare routines, and adopting a lifestyle that promotes calmness and stability. This includes consuming nourishing foods, staying

hydrated, getting enough rest, and engaging in gentle exercise and relaxation techniques.

- It's important to note that Ayurveda takes a holistic approach to health and considers various factors when addressing imbalances. Consulting with an Ayurvedic practitioner can provide personalized guidance and recommendations based on your unique constitution and health needs.

Vata_ yoga suits like hip opening type, improving digestive function, Hip opening yoga poses, such as pigeon pose (Eka

Pada Rajakapotasana) and butterfly pose (Baddha Konasana), are great for increasing flexibility and releasing tension in the hips. These poses can help improve hip mobility, relieve lower back pain, and release emotional stress stored in the hips. Remember to listen to your body, take it slow, and breathe deeply while practicing hip opening yoga poses.

- A brisk walk is a faster-paced form of walking that increases your heart rate and breathing. In Vata Prakriti, a brisk walk helps to ground and stabilize the energy associated with Vata dosha. It can help calm the mind, improve circulation, and promote a sense of balance and stability. By engaging in a brisk walk, Vata individuals can find relief from restlessness and anxiety while enjoying the benefits of physical activity.

Breath work / meditation need to calm anxious mind.

- Pitta dosha (more fire element)_ person having sharp mind, easily get irritated if they become stressed, For individuals with a Pitta constitution in Ayurveda, it is important to focus on maintaining balance and cooling down. They may benefit from practices that promote relaxation, moderation, and a calm environment. This can include incorporating cooling foods, staying hydrated, engaging in gentle exercise,

- In Ayurveda, Pitta dosha is considered to be a precursor of Rakt Dhatu. Rakt Dhatu represents the blood tissue in the body.

- The food we consume plays a crucial role in the formation and quality of Rakt Dhatu. Pitta dosha, responsible for transformation and metabolism, governs the digestion and assimilation of nutrients, which ultimately impacts the formation of Rakt Dhatu.

- When Pitta dosha is in balance, it helps to efficiently digest and absorb nutrients from food, ensuring the production of healthy Rakt Dhatu. However, an imbalance in Pitta dosha can lead to poor digestion, which may affect the quality of Rakt Dhatu and result in various blood-related disorders.

- To maintain a healthy balance of Pitta dosha and support the formation of Rakt Dhatu, Ayurveda recommends following a Pitta-pacifying diet. This includes consuming foods that are cooling, hydrating, and have a sweet, bitter, or astringent taste. Examples of such foods are leafy greens, cucumbers, coconut, barley, and pomegranate.

Pitta-Twisting spine yoga suits (increase detoxification and improve circulation), Spine twisting yoga, also known as Ardha

Matsyendrasana, is a yoga pose that involves twisting the spine. It is beneficial for improving spinal flexibility, toning the abdominal muscles, and stimulating the digestive system. This pose can help relieve tension in the back, neck, and shoulders, and it also helps in detoxifying the body.

Pitta prakriti people are more prone to inflammation bcoz of their difference in microbiome nature in gut, according to recent research each kind of prakriti have different variations of gut microbiome, that's why little variation in one another diet is normal

- Kapha prakriti (Earth and water element)

For someone with a Kapha constitution, it's important to focus on staying active and energized. Incorporate regular exercise, eat lighter foods, and keep a routine to maintain balance.

In Ayurveda, Kapha dosha is considered to be a precursor of all the remaining dhatus except for Rasa (plasma) and Rakt (blood).

Kapha dosha governs stability, structure, and lubrication in the body. It provides the building blocks and nourishment for the formation of the other dhatus, including Mamsa (muscle tissue), Meda (adipose tissue), Asthi (bone tissue), Majja (marrow and nervous tissue), and Shukra

(reproductive tissue).

When Kapha dosha is balanced, it supports the proper formation and functioning of these tissues, promoting strength, stability, and vitality. However, an imbalance in Kapha dosha can lead to excess accumulation and stagnation, which may manifest as issues related to these dhatus.

To maintain a healthy balance of Kapha dosha and support the formation of the remaining dhatus, Ayurveda recommends following a Kapha-pacifying diet and lifestyle. This includes consuming light and warm foods, reducing intake of heavy and oily foods, incorporating spices and herbs with warming properties, and engaging in regular physical activity.

Ayurvedic diet and lifestyle according to season

1. **Sishir**
2. **Vasant** _ kapha prakop kala, pathya _ madhvik sidhu made from fruits Apathya_ heavy food
3. **Grishma ritu/summer season** _ all moisture or sneha in body is absorbed by sun light in summer

Pathya_ cold manth Roasted gram flour sattu is considered beneficial in the summer season in Ayurveda. It has a "sheeta" or cooling effect on the body and laghu light in nature, helping to balance the heat. Sattu is known for its hydrating properties and can help to quench thirst and provide a refreshing boost. It is often consumed as a cooling drink to beat the summer heat and replenish electrolytes., Roasted gram flour sattu is considered a nutritious and cooling food in Ayurveda. It is believed to have a balancing effect on the body, especially during hot seasons. Sattu is known for its high protein content and is often used to make refreshing drinks

Benefits of consuming sattu drink udmanth/roasted gram flour drink

• Sattu is light in nature and good for eye health in summer due to its cooling or light nature, also good for throat health, after vomiting and water loss sattu drink is best to regain water imbalances because sattu drink have property of water retention.

cooling drink, jangal mansras/meat soup, sarkara Sarkara, also known as "sugar" in Ayurveda, is considered to have heating and heavy properties. It is believed to increase Kapha dosha and can be aggravating for certain health conditions. Ayurveda recommends moderation in consuming sugar and suggests using natural sweeteners like jaggery or honey as alternative

Note _ there are certain rules we should know before consuming sattu/roasted gram flour or udmanth drink, we should consume sattu drink after meal good to drink in empty stomach at morning time, we should not consume sattu drink twice a day, it's better to make drink out of sattu instead of making it like dough.

4. Sharad ritu _ **Varsha sanchit pitta is prakupita in Sharad means aggregated pitta dosha in varsha tends to further aggregate in this season,** Excess pitta aggravation can disrupt the delicate balance of the digestive system. It can lead to inflammation and irritation in the digestive tract, which can affect the production and activity of digestive enzymes. The excessive heat and acidity associated with pitta aggravation can impair the functioning of the enzyme-producing cells, leading to a decrease in the production of digestive enzymes. This can result in reduced enzymatic activity and compromised digestion. Balancing pitta through Ayurvedic practices, such as dietary modification can help restore the optimal functioning of digestive enzymes.

Pitta prakop kala pathya food is pitta pacifying foods, pathya food is _ tikt bitter veggies are beneficial to eat Bitter herbs can help stimulate the production of digestive juices, including stomach acid, even in cases of low stomach acid. They can support digestion by promoting the release of enzymes and improving overall digestive functiins, Bitter herbs can help stimulate the production of digestive juices, including stomach acid, even in cases of low stomach acid.

They work by activating bitter receptors in the mouth and digestive system, which in turn triggers a cascade of events that promote the release of digestive enzymes and increase stomach acid secretion. This can help improve digestion and alleviate symptoms associated with low stomach acid.

- tikta sneha/ tikta ghrit which pacify or excrete excess vitiated pitta from blood, Tikta Ghrit, or bitter ghee, is an important formulation in Ayurveda. It is made by combining ghee (clarified butter) with bitter herbs. Tikta Ghrit is believed to have detoxifying properties and is often used to balance Pitta dosha and support liver health. It is also used in Ayurvedic treatments for skin conditions, digestive disorders, and to promote overall well-being. However, it's best to consult with an Ayurvedic practitioner before using Tikta Ghrit to ensure it is appropriate for your specific needs.Tikta Ghrit, or bitter ghee, is an Important formulation in Ayurveda. It is made by combining ghee (clarified butter) with bitter herbs. Tikta Ghrit is believed to have detoxifying properties and is often used to balance Pitta dosha and support liver health. It is also used in Ayurvedic treatments for skin conditions, digestive disorders, and to promote overall well-being. However, it's best to consult with an Ayurvedic practitioner before using tikta ghrit,
- hansoak water _ water charged from Sun than cool down by moon is use to drink in this season. is considered to have special properties in Ayurveda. It is believed that placing water under the moonlight during specific phases can enhance its energy. Hansodak water is thought to have a cooling and calming effect on the body

and mind. It is often used in Ayurvedic rituals and practices to promote balance and well-being. However.

1. Varsha ritu/rainy season _ all three dosas are vitiated, water vipaka turn into Amla rasa, body becomes weak, digestive fire also weak in rainy season.

   Pathya food _ honey mix with water or honey mix with food (madhu sanskarit jala pana or ahar), Honey holds great importance in Ayurveda! It is considered a natural sweetener with various health benefits. Ayurveda views honey as a balancing substance that can help pacify dosha imbalances. It is known for its antimicrobial properties and is often used in Ayurvedic remedies for throat irritation, coughs, and digestive issues. However, it's important to note that honey should not be heated or mixed with hot foods, as it may lose its therapeutic properties. light food

2. Hemant/winter season _ digestive fire enlighten due to traped vayu

Pathya foods_ heavy food, oily or good fat food must include, jentak swedan means using steam room or suana .

Certain foods like curd is advisable in only specific season and contraindicated in others seasons are as follow

Curd_ curd is hot in potency and abhisyandi in nature.Indeed, curd is said to have an "abhisyandi" nature in Ayurveda. This means that it has a tendency to create excessive moisture or phlegm in the body when consumed in large quantities. It's recommended to consume curd in moderation, especially for individuals who have a tendency towards excess phlegm or congestion. Balance is key in

Ayurveda. hemant, shishir, varsha/rainy season, in all these three seasons curd is advisable to consume

Sharad, vasant, grishma (summer season) consumption is contraindicated

- **At night time curd consumption can cause diesease like _ jawarasrkvisarpkusthkamlaAt night time curd consumption can cause diesease like _ jawarasrkvisarpkusthkamla means fever, blood disorder, ersiplias, chronic skin diesease, jaundice so in ayurveda it's advisable to not consume curd at night. According to Ayurveda, eating curd at night may have some disadvantages. It is believed to have a cooling effect on the body, which can disrupt digestion and lead to the formation of toxins. This can potentially cause digestive issues and heaviness in the stomach. It is generally recommended to consume curd during the daytime when digestion is stronger.In Ayurveda, even though curd is considered "hot" in terms of its potency, it can still have a cooling effect on the body after consumption. This cooling effect is believed to be due to its properties and how it interacts with the digestive system. It's important to note that Ayurveda takes into account various factors, including the overall effect of a food item on the body, rather than just its potency.**

Day sleep recommendation according to ayurveda in different seasons

Day sleep is contraindicated in Sharad, Vasant, varsha (rainy season)

In Ayurveda, day sleep, also known as "Divaswapna, " is generally not recommended. It is believed to disturb the natural balance of the doshas, particularly Kapha dosha, leading to lethargy, heaviness, and digestive issues. However, there may be specific circumstances or health conditions where a short nap during the day can be beneficial.

Day sleep is contraindicated in some seasons because it can aggravate certain doshas, disrupt the body's natural rhythms, and lead to sluggishness. It's best to align your sleep schedule with the natural cycle of the day and night for optimal energy and well-being.

Season in which it's advisable to avoid

Sunlight or dew drops

Sharad and varsha (rainy season) Aatap sunlight or dew drops is contraindicated and should be avoided.

Sunlight is avoided in specific seasons in Ayurveda because excessive sun exposure during certain times can lead to imbalances in the doshas and cause heat-related issues. Ayurveda suggests being mindful of the intensity of the sun and taking necessary precautions to protect oneself, such as seeking shade, wearing protective clothing, and using natural sunscreens. It's all about maintaining a balance and keeping the body in harmony with the environment.

Psychosomatic diesease in morden time and it's cure and prevention through ayurveda

- Psychosomatic diseases are conditions that are influenced by both psychological and physical factors. They occur when emotional or mental stressors manifest as physical symptoms or illnesses. Examples include psoriasis, where stress can trigger or worsen flare-ups, and irritable bowel syndrome, where stress can exacerbate digestive symptoms. It's important to address both the psychological and physical aspects of these conditions for holistic healing.

Psychosomatic diseases are conditions in which emotional or mental factors play a significant role in causing or worsening physical symptoms. These symptoms can include pain, fatigue, digestive issues, skin problems, and more. The mind-body connection is important in understanding and managing these diseases, as addressing the underlying psychological factors can help alleviate the physical symptoms. It's a fascinating field that highlights the intricate relationship between our thoughts, emotions, and physical well-being.

In ayurveda Nasya procedure can treat 90percent of diesease by it's calming and detoxifying action on brain

In Ayurveda, nasya is a therapeutic practice that involves administering herbal oils or medicated substances through the nasal passages. While nasya is commonly used for various conditions like sinus congestion and allergies, it may also have a positive impact on psychosomatic diseases. The nasal passages are considered a gateway to the mind, and nasya helps balance the doshas, calm the mind, and promote overall well-being.

- There are several types of nasya in Ayurveda, each with its own specific purpose and benefits. Some common types include Pratimarsh Nasya, which is done daily for general maintenance; Brihmana Nasya, which nourishes and strengthens the nasal passages; Shamana Nasya, which pacifies doshic imbalances; and Marsha Nasya, which involves forceful administration of medicated oils. Each type of nasya has its own unique techniques and uses.

- Partimarsh nasya which is done daily is good to practice in daily rituals

Procedure of partimarsh nasya

1. **Roll** a towel and put it under the neck
2. **Massage nose and sinuses area** if possible can steam before nasya
3. **Put** your neck under rolled towel and instill 2 drop of Anu oil in each nostrils
4. Spit out the mucus comes in mouth after Nasya • **Benefits of nasya**

Nasya in Ayurveda is an amazing therapy with many benefits! It involves the administration of medicated oils or powders into the nostrils. This helps to clear the nasal passages, relieve sinus congestion, and improve respiratory health. Nasya also has a positive impact on mental clarity and can promote overall well-being. It's a wonderful way to support your health.

Treatment protocol in Ayurveda and its understanding in depth

- **In Ayurveda, treatment protocols are personalized based on an individual's unique constitution, imbalances, and specific health concerns. It typically involves a combination of dietary and lifestyle recommendations, herbal remedies, detoxification procedures, and therapeutic practices like yoga and meditation.**

- In Ayurveda, the seven tissues, known as dhatus, are described as the building blocks of the body. They include rasa (plasma), rakta (blood), mamsa (muscle), meda (fat), asthi (bone), majja (bone marrow), and shukra (reproductive tissue). Each dhatu has its own unique qualities and functions, and they work together to maintain overall health and well-being.

- the seven dhatus (tissues) are described as the fundamental components of the human body. Each dhatu has its own specific functions and characteristics. Rasa nourishes the body and provides fluidity, rakta carries oxygen and nutrients, mamsa provides structure and movement, meda stores energy, asthi supports the body's framework, majja nourishes the nervous system, and shukra is responsible for reproduction. These dhatus work together to maintain overall health and balance in the body.

- in Ayurveda, there is a correlation between the Pancha Mahabhutas (five elements) and the Dhatus (tissues) in the body. Each Dhatu is associated with a specific Mahabhuta. Ras Dhatu, which represents the plasma and lymphatic system, is prominently associated with the Jala Mahabhuta (water element). This understanding helps in identifying imbalances and finding ways to restore harmony within the body.

- the formation of the seven dhatus (tissues) involves a sequential process. Each dhatu is formed from the previous one, starting with rasa (plasma) and progressing through rakta (blood), mamsa (muscle), meda (fat), asthi (bone), majja (bone marrow), and finally shukra (reproductive tissue). As for the updhatu, there are specific ones related to certain body parts. Artav is the updhatu of Rasa(plasma)and is associated with the menstrual cycle. Kesh refers to the updhatu of asthi and represents the hair tissue. Nakh corresponds to the updhatu of asthi as well and refers to the nails. These updhatu play important roles in their respective body parts and contribute to overall health and well-being.

  Note_ updhatu can be understood by byproduct, so here for maintenance of hair and nail proper nourishment of each dhatu especially asthi dhatu (bones) is essential.In Ayurveda, updhatu refers to the byproducts or secondary tissues that are formed as a result of the metabolism and transformation of the main dhatus. For example, the updhatu of Rasa is artav, which is associated with the menstrual cycle. Kesh and nakh are also considered updhatu, related to the asthi (bone) tissue, representing hair and nails respectively. These updhatu play specific roles in their respective body parts and contribute to overall health and balance according to Ayurvedic principles.

- **According to Ayurveda, the formation of each dhatu (tissue) takes a specific amount of time. Rasa (plasma) is formed in 5 days, rakta (blood) in 10 days, mamsa (muscle) in 15 days, meda (fat) in 20 days, asthi (bone) in 25 days, majja (bone marrow) in 30 days, and shukra**

(reproductive tissue) in 35 days. These timeframes represent the approximate duration it takes for each dhatu to develop fully.

Note _ formation of muscles takes 15 day if a patient suffering from chronic pain in muscles it takes almost 15 day to get proper results with medicine or herbs that's why Agni karma a ayurvedic procedure is done for instant relief from pain.

Agni karma in Ayurveda refers to a therapeutic procedure involving the application of heat or fire to specific points on the body. It is used to alleviate pain, reduce inflammation, and promote healing. Agni karma is believed to stimulate blood flow, improve circulation, and balance the doshas. This procedure is typically performed using a heated instrument or herbal preparations. It is important to consult with a qualified Ayurvedic practitioner before

undergoing any Ayurvedic treatments

In blood disorder with medication it will take almost 10 days to show results through herbs and formulation so

for instant relief jaloka or cupping therapy is done to get instant relief

Cupping therapy is also sunnah in Islam

Jaloka treatment, also known as leech therapy, is a traditional Ayurvedic treatment method. It involves the application of medicinal leeches to the body to extract impure blood and promote healing. Jaloka treatment is believed to improve blood circulation, reduce inflammation, and detoxify the body. It is commonly used for conditions such as skin disorders, joint pain, and certain circulatory issues. However,

Jaloka treatment, also known as leech therapy, is a traditional Ayurvedic treatment method. It involves the application of medicinal leeches to the body to extract impure blood and promote healing. Jaloka treatment is believed to improve blood circulation, reduce inflammation, and detoxify the body. It is commonly used for conditions such as skin disorders, joint pain, and certain circulatory issues.

In Ayurveda, cupping therapy is a therapeutic technique that involves placing cups on the skin to create suction. This suction helps to stimulate blood flow, relieve muscle tension, and promote healing. Cupping is used to address various conditions like pain, inflammation, and respiratory issues.

Dhatu tissue kshay vridhi lakshan, tissue depletion symptoms

- **Muscle depletion can contribute to joint pain due to the changes it causes in the body's physiology. When muscles weaken or atrophy, it can lead to imbalances in joint stability and support. This can put additional stress on the joints, leading to pain and discomfort.**

Additionally, decreased muscle mass can result in reduced cushioning and shock absorption, further exacerbating joint pain. Muscle loss can contribute to the looseness of Dhamni (blood vessels) in Ayurveda through various physiological mechanisms. When muscles weaken, they provide less support and stability to the blood vessels, which can lead to their relaxation and increased laxity. This can result in reduced tone and integrity of the blood vessel walls, potentially affecting blood flow and circulation. It is important to maintain muscle strength through regular exercise and a balanced diet to support the health and integrity of the Dhamni system.

- Rakt kshay, or blood loss, can contribute to sira saithilya, which means vessel looseness in Ayurveda. When there is significant blood loss, it can lead to a decrease in blood volume and a reduction in the nutrients and oxygen being delivered to the tissues. This can weaken the vessel walls and cause them to become loose or lax. It is important to address and treat the underlying cause of blood loss and support the body's ability to regenerate blood cells and maintain healthy blood vessels.
- When there is a loss of fat (meda) tissue in the joints, it can lead to sandhi sphutan (joint instability) and crepitation. This can occur due to the reduced cushioning and lubrication provided by the fat tissue, causing the joint surfaces to rub against each other, resulting in cracking or popping sounds. It's important to address this issue to prevent further joint damage and discomfort. Ayurvedic treatments aim to strengthen the joints, promote healthy fat tissue, and improve joint stability.

- Loss of fat (meda) tissue in the joints can lead to sandhi sunyata (joint emptiness) and sucking pain. This occurs when the cushioning and lubrication provided by the fat tissue are reduced, causing the joint surfaces to have less support and resulting in a sensation of emptiness and a sucking pain.
- Loss of asthi (bone) tissue can contribute to sandhi (joint) looseness and depletion. When the bones become weak or depleted, it can affect the stability and strength of the joints, leading to joint looseness and instability. It's important to address this issue to prevent further joint damage and discomfort.
- Loss of majja (marrow) tissue can contribute to bone emptiness or sucking pain. Majja is responsible for providing nourishment and support to the bones. When there is depletion or loss of majja, it can lead to a sensation of emptiness in the bones and cause sucking pain. This can result in discomfort and instability in the affected areas.
- In Ayurveda, kriyakala refers to the specific time or period during which a particular treatment or procedure is performed. It takes into account the individual's constitution, the nature of the ailment, and the external environment. The timing of treatments is believed to align with the natural rhythms of the body and its doshas, optimizing the therapeutic effects. By considering the physiological state of the body at different times, Ayurveda aims to enhance the efficacy of treatments and support the body's innate healing processes.

Kriyakala refers to the seven stages of disease progression in Ayurveda. These stages are:

1. Sanchaya (Accumulation): The initial stage where the doshas start accumulating in the body.

In Ayurveda, during the Sanchay Avastha stage, the doshas accumulate in their respective places in the body. For example, Vata accumulates below the navel, Kapha accumulates above the clavicle, and in terms of the Dhatu (tissue) level, Asthi Dhatu is accumulated by vata dosha

During this stage, the desire to eat foods that are opposite to the aggravated dosha or the accumulated substance is common. This helps to balance the doshas and support overall wellbeing. It's fascinating how Ayurveda focuses on understanding the body's natural processes and finding ways to restore balance.

2. Prakopa (Aggravation): The doshas become aggravated and start spreading throughout the body.

Vata prakop symptoms are needdle pricking pain in abdomen Oh, I totally get what you mean! Needle pricking pain in the abdomen can be a symptom of Vata aggravation. In Ayurveda, Vata imbalances can cause digestive discomfort and pain. It's important to nurture your Vata dosha by following a Vata-pacifying diet and lifestyle. Warm, cooked foods, gentle exercise like yoga, and staying hydrated can help balance Vata.

Pitta prakop symptoms are belching with sour taste, indigestion, thrist, burn Oh, I totally understand what you're talking about! Belching with a sour taste, indigestion, thirst, and a burning sensation can be symptoms of Pitta aggravation. In Ayurveda, Pitta imbalances can lead to these discomforts. To balance Pitta, it's recommended to incorporate cooling foods like

cucumber, coconut water, and sweet fruits. Avoiding spicy and fried foods can also be helpful. Additionally, practicing stress-reducing activities like meditation and yoga can support overall balance.

Kapha prakop symptoms are anorexia, nausea, Oh, Anorexia and nausea can be symptoms of Kapha aggravation. In Ayurveda, Kapha imbalances can affect digestion and lead to these discomforts. It's important to balance Kapha by incorporating warm and light foods into your diet, such as ginger, spices, and bitter greens. Regular exercise, especially cardio activities, can also help stimulate digestion and balance Kapha.

3. Prasara (Spread): The aggravated doshas spread to different parts of the body, causing symptoms in kapha prasar like anorexia, indigestion, bodyach, vomiting (arochakavipakaangsaad chardi)

Vata prasar vimarggaman, gud gud sound in stomach also sign of weak digestive fire, Oh, When there's a gud gud sound in the stomach, it can be a sign of weak digestive fire. In Ayurveda, it's believed that imbalanced Vata dosha can affect digestion and cause such sounds. Taking care of your digestive fire is important for overall health. Have you tried CCF tea? It's an Ayurvedic herbal blend of cumin, coriander, and fennel seeds that can help support digestion. And help in vata nigrah or alleviate excess vata

Pitta prasar heatying drying burning sensation Oh, When Pitta dosha is imbalanced, it can cause a heating, drying, and burning sensation in the body. It can be quite uncomfortable! In Ayurveda, it's recommended to balance Pitta by incorporating cooling and soothing

practices. Drinking coconut water, eating juicy fruits like watermelon, and applying cooling oils like coconut oil can help alleviate those sensations.

In the Prasara Avastha stage of Kriya Kala, the doshas can become imbalanced and vata dosha may get vitiated in the sakha (peripheral) tissues, away from the kostha (gastrointestinal tract). To address this, Ayurveda suggests activities like vishyandan (vilayan), srotosodhan (channel cleansing)and vata nigrah (calming excess vata dosha) through the use of vatanashak medications. These medications aim to restore balance and harmony to the body.

Note_ before locatization of doshas (kha vaigunya in srotas) means channel of body get affected by doshas for example vata dosha makes channel dry or irritates it further cause easy lodgement of aggrevated Dosha in channels

For easy understanding if channel of body get affected by vata or pitta it looses it's natural shape or property breakdown in different channels

Of organ causes obstruction or any other systems

So that normal circulation may get affected because of changes in natural property and can provide breakdown spaces of lodgement of toxins and can cause 4 th stage of kriyakala which is sthan samshray

Note _ During the dosha Sanchay, the doshas can spread throughout the body via the blood, leading to the sthan samshraya . Bloodletting therapy or cupping therapy can indeed be beneficial during the Sanchay Avastha stage. These therapies help to remove excess doshas and

promote the flow of energy, ultimately supporting the body's natural healing process.

6. Sthana Samshraya (Localization) purvarupa/ prodomal syndrome: specifically dosha dusya samurchana occur here means dosa or toxin get mix with dushya or tissue, The doshas localize in a specific channel (srotas) area or organ, leading to more specific symptoms, When there is strotos (channel) obstruction in Ayurveda, During this stage, the doshas start to accumulate in specific locations or sthanas in the body. This accumulation can lead to the manifestation of early signs and symptoms that indicate an imbalance or impending illness Sthansansray in kriya kala is stage of purvarupa or prodromal syndrome (early sign) . These signs and symptoms can vary depending on the specific dosha involved. It's important to recognize these early indicators and take appropriate measures to restore balance and prevent the progression of the doshic imbalance. Ayurveda offers various approaches, such as dietary adjustments, lifestyle modifications.

Note_ in prasar avastha of kriyakala this stage drugs causing srotas or channel cleansing or sroto sodhan ausadhi should be given like, for example_ gugglu, triphala by clearing channels of body circulation improve or lodgement to toxins expels out.

Or in this stage in chronic issues like autoimmune skin diesease or any chronic diesease panchkarma therapy is good specifically Virechana procedure is beneficial Virechana is a process in Ayurveda that focuses on cleansing and purifying the body's channels of elimination, including the digestive tract and the liver. It

involves the administration of specific herbs and formulations to induce a controlled purgation, eliminating toxins and excess Pitta from the body. This process aims to restore balance and promote overall well-being. It is typically performed under the guidance of an Ayurvedic practitioner.

7. Vyakti (Manifestation): The disease becomes fully manifested with clear signs and symptoms.

In this stage generally kasay kalpana is beneficial Kasay, or herbal decoctions, are an integral part of Ayurveda. They are made by boiling specific herbs in water to extract their medicinal properties. Kasay is often used to treat various health conditions and imbalances in the body. These decoctions can be tailored to individual needs and dosha imbalances, making them a versatile and effective form of Ayurvedic treatment. Whether it's for boosting immunity, promoting digestion, or addressing specific health concerns, kasay plays a significant role in Ayurvedic healing.

Kasay, or herbal decoctions, possess unique properties based on the herbs used. They can have a wide range of effects on the body, such as promoting digestion, boosting immunity, reducing inflammation, detoxifying the body, and balancing the doshas. The specific properties of a kasay depend on the herbs included in the formulation. Ayurvedic practitioners carefully select herbs to create kasay that target specific health concerns and imbalances. It's important to consult with an Ayurvedic expert to determine the most appropriate kasay for your individual needs.

Along with kasay pH balancing or making body alkaline through ayurvedic medicine is also necessary as per requirement In Ayurveda, there are various treatments and practices that aim to balance the pH levels in the body. These treatments focus on restoring the body's natural equilibrium by incorporating specific herbs, dietary changes, and lifestyle modifications.

8. Bheda (Diversification): The disease starts affecting different tissues and organs, leading to complications.in this stage generally panchkarma is prescribed like swedan treatment Swedana, or Ayurvedic sweating therapy, is an important treatment in Ayurveda. It involves inducing sweat to eliminate toxins, improve circulation, and promote relaxation. There are different methods of swedana, such as steam therapy, herbal poultices, and warm oil massages. These treatments help to open up the channels of the body, allowing for the release of toxins and balancing the doshas. Swedana can be beneficial for various conditions, including muscle stiffness, joint pain, respiratory issues, and stress. It's best to consult with an Ayurvedic practitioner to determine the most suitable swedana treatment for your specific needs.

Note _ in arthritis generally baluka swedana is prescribed Baluka Swedana, also known as poultice sweating, is a type of swedana treatment in Ayurveda. It involves applying warm herbal poultices to specific areas of the body to induce sweating and promote therapeutic benefits. The poultices are made by combining herbs with a heating agent, such as sand, rice, or salt, and then applying them to the body. The heat from the poultices helps to open up the channels, improve circulation, and relieve muscle tension and joint pain. Baluka Swedana is often used in combination with other Ayurvedic

treatments to enhance their effectiveness. It's best to consult with an Ayurvedic practitioner to determine if Baluka Swedana is suitable for your specific needs.

7. Upashaya (Resolution): The disease either resolves on its own or with the help of treatment.

It's important to note that Ayurvedic treatment aims to intervene at the early stages to prevent the progression of the disease.

• Sthaniya chikitsa in Ayurveda refers to localized or specific treatment approaches. It involves targeting a specific area or organ of the body for therapeutic interventions. This can include various Ayurvedic treatments such as herbal applications, oil massages, and specific dietary recommendations.

To understand treatment of specific organ or area of body first we need to understand Dosha distribution according to part of body According to Ayurveda, Vata, Pitta, and Kapha are present in different parts of the body. Vata is predominant in the lower part of the body, including the colon, hips, and legs.

Pitta is mainly located in the middle part of the body, such as the small intestine, liver, and stomach. Kapha is primarily present in the upper part of the body, including the chest, lungs, and head. Balancing these doshas in their respective areas is important for maintaining overall health and well-being.

According to Ayurveda, Vata, Pitta, and Kapha are present in all parts and organs of the body. However, each dosha has a predominant influence on certain areas. Vata is primarily associated with the nervous system and

governs movement and communication. Pitta is mainly located in the digestive system, liver, and metabolism. Kapha is centered in the respiratory system, joints, and mucous membranes. It's important to maintain balance among the three doshas for overall well-being.

The factors of country, time, season, and Individual constitution play a significant role in disease treatment in Ayurveda. Localized treatment, known as "sthaniya chikitsa, " is also emphasized. Ayurveda considers these factors to create a personalized and effective approach to healing.

In sthaniya chikitsa for example if there is a diesease of upper respiratory system that for upper respiratory system predominant dosha is kapha so before treating upper respiratory problems first we need to pay attention on basis factor affecting predominant dosha which is Desh, kala(time), season, individual constitution

If all these 4 factor aggrevate predominant dosha than we should treat sthaniya organ according to it's predominant dosha which is kapha in upper respiratory problems

If these 4 factor are not similar to predominant dosha than treatment should be based on vitiated Dosha like for in cough or kasa vata dosha is vitiated than first we treat vata and kapha which is sthaniya dosha.

Tissues (dhatu)dosha, vikriti or it's symptoms and treatment

9. Rasadhatu dusti symptoms are

Ras pardosaj vikara is a term used in Ayurveda to describe disorders related to rasa or first tissue of body formed just after meal or digestion/the digestion and metabolism of the bodily tissues. It refers to the improper functioning of the digestive fire (agni) and the accumulation of toxins (ama) in the body. This can lead to various health issues. Ayurveda recommends balancing the doshas through diet, lifestyle, and herbal remedies to promote optimal digestion and overall well-being.

in Ayurveda to describe the condition of "Dust Rasaj Rog" or disorders caused by the imbalance of the Rasa doshas. It manifests with symptoms like anorexia, heaviness in the body, body ache, fever, lethargy, dizziness, anemia and more. Ayurvedic treatments focus on restoring the balance of the doshas through herbal remedies, dietary modifications, is langhan

That's interesting! Ayurveda offers various methods for balancing the rasa Dhatu doshas, and Langan is one of them. The ten types you mentioned include techniques like fasting (Upvas), exercise (Vayam), and therapies like Vaman (emesis) and Virechan (purgation), sunbath in morning, vayu Sevan, fasting mainly dry fasting, hebs having pachan or digestive nature like ginger, trikatu etc Each method has its unique benefits in promoting overall well-being. It's always best to consult with an Ayurvedic practitioner for personalized advice.

10. Raktasrog refers to the imbalance or vikriti in the blood, which can manifest as various skin disorders like vitiligo and psoriasis. blood disorders, or "raktas rog" in

Ayurveda. These disorders, such as hemorrhoids (raktpit), skin conditions like vitiligo (svitra), and others, are considered as imbalances or “vikrti” in the blood (“dosht rakta”). Ayurveda offers treatments and remedies to address these conditions. Ayurveda focuses on treating these conditions by addressing the root cause and restoring balance in the body.

Blood disorders, or Rakta Vikritis, can be addressed through various therapies in Ayurveda. Blood cooling herbs(Vasa,), virechana therapy, fasting, and Rakta Vishravarna (bloodletting therapies) are commonly used treatments. These therapies aim to restore balance in the blood and promote overall well-being. It’s important to consult with an Ayurvedic practitioner for a detailed description and guidance on the appropriate use of these therapies for specific blood disorders.

• In Ayurveda, there are various types of Kalpana, which are specific methods of preparing and administering herbal medicines. These methods help enhance the therapeutic effects of the herbs. Here are a few types of Kalpana and their uses:

2. Kashaya (Decoction): This involves boiling the herbs in water to extract their medicinal properties. Kashayas are commonly used for internal consumption to treat various ailments.

3. Churna (Powder): Herbs are dried and powdered, either individually or in combinations. Churna is often taken with warm water or honey to aid digestion and promote overall wellbeing.Churna in Ayurveda is known for its aptarpana (depleting) or tikshna (sharp) properties. These properties make churna formulations

effective in promoting detoxification, eliminating ama (toxins), and balancing the doshas.

Aptarpana property refers to the ability of churna to remove excess doshas and ama from the body, supporting the cleansing and purification processes. This property helps in alleviating conditions related to accumulation or stagnation of doshas, improving digestion, and promoting overall wellness.

Tikshna property refers to the sharpness or penetrating nature of churna. This quality allows churna to penetrate deep into the tissues and channels of the body, enhancing its therapeutic effects. Tikshna churna formulations are particularly beneficial in conditions where there is a need for deeper cleansing and rejuvenation.

Bhasma or minerals preparation in ayurveda

- Bhasma or mineral preparations in Ayurveda are considered both rasayan (rejuvenating) and lekhana (scraping) in nature.

- Rasayan refers to the ability of bhasma to nourish and rejuvenate the body, promoting longevity, vitality, and overall well-being. Bhasma preparations are believed to enhance cellular function, strengthen the immune system, and support the body's natural healing processes.

- On the other hand, lekhana refers to the scraping or cleansing action of bhasma. Certain bhasma preparations are used to eliminate toxins, metabolic waste, and accumulated ama from the body. This scraping action helps in purifying the tissues, improving digestion, and promoting healthy metabolism.

- It is important to note that bhasma preparations should always be taken under the guidance of a qualified Ayurvedic practitioner, as they involve a specialized process of purification and preparation to ensure their safety and efficacy.

4. Vati (Tablets): Herbs are powdered and combined with binding agents to form tablets. Vati is a convenient and easy way of taking herbal medicines, especially for those who prefer not to consume powders or liquids.Vati kalpana is a method of preparing herbal medicines in the form of tablets. In this process, herbs are finely powdered and mixed with binding agents such as ghee, honey, or jaggery. The mixture is then rolled into small tablets. Vati is a convenient and easy way to consume herbal rcmedies as it eliminates the need for measuring and mixing powders. These tablets can be easily swallowed with water or honey. Vati kalpana allows for precise dosing and prolonged shelf life of the herbal medicines. It is commonly used in Ayurveda for various purposes, including promoting digestion, balancing doshas .

examples of Kharliye Rasayan, like Gandhak Rasayan and Arogyavardhini vati Gandhak Rasayan is an Ayurvedic preparation that involves grinding sulfur (gandhak) into a fine powder using a mortar and pestle. It is known for its detoxifying and purifying properties and is often used to support healthy skin and respiratory health.

Arogyavardhini is another Ayurvedic Rasayana that may involve grinding various herbs and minerals together in a mortar and pestle. It is believed to promote overall well-being and support the digestive system, liver health, and metabolism. Kharliye Rasayan, being heavy in nature, is often used in Ayurveda to address diseases that have a spreading nature, such as rheumatoid arthritis (Amavata) and autoimmune diseases like psoriasis. These rasayanas are formulated to balance the body and help manage the symptoms of these conditions.

However, it's important to note that due to their heavy nature,

Kharliye Rasayanas can sometimes have side effects such as diarrhea and a weakened digestive fire. This is why it's essential to take them under the guidance of an experienced Ayurvedic practitioner who can tailor the dosage and monitor any potential adverse effects.

5. Asava and Arishta (Fermented Formulations): These are herbal liquids created by fermenting herbs with sugars, honey, or jaggery. Asava and Arishta are known for their digestive and rejuvenating properties.

6. Ghrita (Medicated Ghee): Ghee is prepared by simmering herbs in clarified butter. Ghrita is used for various purposes, such as improving digestion, nourishing the body, and balancing doshas.

7. Taila (Medicated Oil): Herbs are infused in oils through a process of heating and cooling. Taila is commonly used for external application, such as in massage therapies and to alleviate joint and muscle pain.

These are just a few examples of the different types of Kalpana used in Ayurveda. Each method has its own unique benefits and uses, depending on the specific herbs and the desired therapeutic effects.

Marma points and maneuver for organ reset

Marma points for digestive problems

In Ayurveda, marma points are vital energy points in the bodyMarma In Ayurveda, these junctions are considered to be vital energy centers where various channels and pathways intersect. By working on these junctions, practitioners aim to balance the flow of energy and promote overall well-being. . For digestive problems, the following marma points can be beneficial:

For instant relief pressing these points for 9 times

1. Hridaya (heart) marma point: Located at the center of the chest, massaging this point can help balance digestion and promote a healthy appetite.
2. Nabhi (navel) marma point: Found around the navel area, stimulating this point can improve digestion, relieve bloating, and support overall gastrointestinal health.
3. Vamana (vomiting reflex) marma point: Situated on the back of the neck, gently applying pressure to this point can help alleviate nausea, vomiting, and indigestion.
4. Hand marma or vital points use in plihaudar spleendiesease, kidney diesease vrikudar description In Ayurveda, the specific names of the hand marma points are as follows:
    1. Manibandha Marma
    2. Hasti Marma
    3. Adhipati Marma
    4. Sandhi Marma

5. Mushtika Marma
6. Katakamukha Marma

These are just a few examples. There are several more marma points on the hands with unique

Face marma to relieve nasal blockage

- To relieve nose blockage, you can try stimulating the Marma points associated with the nasal area. One such Marma point is called "phana Marma, " Gently massaging or applying gentle pressure to this point may help alleviate nasal congestion. "phana Marma" is located on either side of the nostrils. Stimulating these points may also provide relief.
- The Shringatak Marma, also known as the Face Marma, is a significant Marma point located on the face below cheek bone at nasolobial fold . It is associated with various facial muscles and is believed to have an impact on the overall health and appearance of the face. Stimulating

this Marma point through gentle massage or pressure can help promote circulation, relieve tension, and enhance the natural glow of the skin and also relieve nasal blockage

1. Fascia maneuver or marma therapy

- **The fascia maneuver refers to a technique used in physical therapy to release tension and improve mobility in the fascia, the connective tissue that surrounds muscles and organs. It involves applying gentle pressure and stretching to specific areas of the body to help alleviate pain and improve function.**

Throughout evolution our body's fascia or muscle is still design in same way as before but our lifestyle evolve we started using plane surface for walking and doing our daily routine but

our ancestors during initial days of evolution use to walk on rocks or uneven surfaces this is how our muscles or fascia designed to do daily activities, According to recent studies, walking on plains may not provide the same benefits as walking on stones. Walking on uneven surfaces, such as stones, can engage more muscles, improve balance, and enhance proprioception. This can help strengthen the muscles and joints, promote better posture, and increase overall stability. However, it's important to find a balance and incorporate a variety of walking surfaces into your routine to reap the benefits of both.

In recent studies in patients of depression walking on rocks for 30 minutes reduce their symptoms of depression and help improve quality of life or Walking barefoot can have several benefits! It allows for better sensory feedback, strengthens the muscles in your feet and legs, and can improve balance and posture. Plus, it's a great way to connect with nature and feel grounded, Walking barefoot on grass can be a delightful experience! It allows you to connect with nature, feel the softness of the grass beneath your feet, and enjoy the sensation of being grounded. Plus, it can provide a refreshing break from wearing shoes and give your feet a chance to breathe.

This practice is a kind of reflexology is common in china Where it's called "tap shek"and government encourages construction of cablestone footpath to improve fitness and overall health.

Acupressure slippers /rock sleepers may also help target the nerve endings as result, better circulation and relaxed nerve induce better sleep and relief foot pain.

In Ayurveda it's recommended to do padabhayang/ foot massage with kansa (metal) before bed it helps improve sleep and memory

Practically if we see the reasons behind padabhayang or foot massage is our feet has largest pores in the body medicated oils get easily absorbed in feet and shoots our nervous system quickly.

2. Fascia maneuver for face

Nowadays using kansa on face or quartz also help reduce inflammation and water retention, expel toxins out of undereye area

- In Ayurveda, Marma points are specific energy points in the body that can be stimulated to promote healing and relieve pain. For lower back pain, there are a few Marma points that can be targeted. Gentle massage or applying pressure to this point may help alleviate discomfort.

- Important marma points for lower back pain

1. Katikatarun Marma is a specific Marma point in Ayurveda that is located in the lower back region. It is situated near the sacrum and the area where the spine meets the pelvis. Stimulating this Marma point through gentle massage or applying pressure may help alleviate discomfort and promote balance in the lower back region.
2. Nitamb Marma is a specific Marma point in Ayurveda that is located in the buttock region. It is situated in the

area where the gluteal muscles meet the pelvic bone. Stimulating this Marma point through gentle massage or applying pressure may help alleviate discomfort and promote balance in the buttock area.

3. Parsavsandhi Marma refers to the junction points of Marma in the body. These junctions can be found at various locations where different Marma points meet. The specific locations of Parsavsandhi Marma can vary its position is at level of elbow joint on back side.
4. The Gulph Marma is a significant Marma point located in the ankle region. It is situated where the bones of the lower leg meet the bones of the foot. Stimulating this Marma point can help improve circulation, relieve pain, and promote balance in the ankle area.
5. Kshipra marma _ location in web between thumb and fingure

• Fascia maneuver for internal soft organ In Ayurveda Bandh is given in yogic practices

Especially mula bandh is for lower internal soft organs in modern Era it can be understand by using term kegal exercise, kegel exercises are great for strengthening the pelvic floor muscles! They can help with bladder control and sexual health.

Mula bandh technique

Mula Bandh is a yogic practice that involves engaging and contracting the pelvic floor muscles. It can help improve focus, stability, and energy flow.

- Inhale deeply and hold the breath almost for 5 second also lift the muscles of pelvic floor

- Concentrate on muladhara chakra and firmly contract anal muscles
- hold the muscular contraction for almost 10 second and breath as long as possible and comfortable with long exhalation
- With long exhalation almost for 5 second retain the starting position lower the muscles of pelvic floor then breath normally in this position for sometime

Benefits of mula Bandh

- help strengthen pelvic floor
- relief hemmoroids and congestion in pelvic area
- Relief in urine incontinence / urinary infection
- In males increase sperm count, sperm motility (fertility) .

General tips for overall wellness

1.We should not drink water after meal for atleast 1 hrs, only buttermilk, lemonade can boost digestive enzymes and we can consume after meal bcoz food generally collect in jathar/stomach/duodenum stomach acid can be diluted by water and impair digestion which inturn results in gas, bloating

Drinking 30 min before meal or 1 hrs after meal is good for digestion.

2. In morning right after wake up drinking water atleast 2_3 glass help in elimination of toxins

- Drink water slowly once in atleast 3sip the saliva(alkaline) neutalize excess acid in stomach inturn reduce burning, hyperacidity
- According to recent studies, adopting alkaline habits can help reduce the risk of hyperacidity. Drinking water sip by sip is one such habit that can help maintain a balanced pH level in the body and prevent excessive acidity.
- Drinking water sip by sip can have several benefits. It allows for better hydration as it helps the body absorb water more efficiently. It also promotes mindful drinking, helping you stay aware of your water intake throughout the day. Sipping water slowly can also aid digestion and prevent overhydration. Overall, it's a good practice to stay hydrated and listen to your body's needs.

In depth for better understanding if stomach

Amlata/toxin/acidity neutalize simultaneously blood acidity also get neutralize and prevent many skin issues or balance tridosha in body

1. After morning breakfast citrus fruit juice, after lunch buttermilk, after dinner milk is good for digestion and overall health.
2. According to recent studies, incorporating alkaline habits into your lifestyle can promote overall wellness. This includes consuming a diet rich in fruits and vegetables, staying hydrated, practicing stress management techniques, getting regular exercise, and prioritizing quality sleep. These habits can help maintain a balanced pH level in the body and support optimal health.
3. arsenic and mercury present in cosmetic products can indeed cause adrenal and endocrine disruption. These toxic substances can interfere with hormone production, signaling, and overall endocrine function, leading to imbalances and potential health issues. It's important to be mindful of the ingredients in cosmetic products and choose safer alternatives.Regular frequency of meals and snacks can support adrenal health by providing a steady supply of nutrients and preventing blood sugar fluctuations. This helps to regulate cortisol levels and support adrenal function. It's important to maintain a balanced diet and manage stress for overall adrenal health.
4. mercury, cadmium, and arsenic have been identified as endocrine disruptors in research studies. They can interfere with the normal functioning of hormones in the

body. These substances can disrupt the endocrine system by mimicking or blocking hormones, affecting hormone production, and interfering with hormone signaling pathways. This can lead to various health issues and imbalances in the body, incorporating vitamin C in your diet can help mitigate the side effects of mercury and reduce the risk of endocrine disruption. Vitamin C acts as an antioxidant and helps in detoxifying harmful substances like mercury from the body.Vitamin C helps support adrenal health by playing a crucial role in the production of cortisol, a hormone released by the adrenal glands. It also acts as an antioxidant, helping to reduce oxidative stress and support overall adrenal function. Including vitamin C-rich foods in your diet, such as citrus fruits, strawberries, and bell peppers, can be beneficial for adrenal health.

5. Yavagu is a type of Ayurvedic therapeutic gruel that is commonly used for detoxification and to balance the body after an acidic state or any animal bite. It is prepared by boiling rice or barley with water until it becomes a smooth porridge-like consistency. Yavagu helps to soothe the digestive system, eliminate toxins, and restore the body's natural balance. It can be beneficial in supporting the healing process after an acidic body condition or an animal bite.Yavagu is typically made by boiling rice or barley with water until it reaches a porridge-like consistency. The exact composition of Yavagu water may vary depending on the specific recipe or ingredients used. It is commonly prepared by simmering one part rice or barley with six /6parts water. The mixture is cooked until the grains are soft and the water has thickened. Yavagu can be flavored

with spices or herbs according to personal preference. It is a nourishing and detoxifying dish in Ayurveda.

6. Sure, here are some general marma points that are believed to promote overall wellness:

- Minimum 9 times pressing /Stimulating these Marma points gives instant relief

    1. Sthapani: Located in the center of the forehead, between the eyebrows. It is associated with calming the mind and relieving stress.
    2. Hridaya: Found in the center of the chest, near the heart. Stimulating this point is believed to promote emotional balance and heart health.
    3. Nabhi: Located around the navel area. It is associated with digestion and can help improve gut health.
    4. Kshipra: Found on the back of the neck, at the base of the skull. Stimulating this point may help relieve tension and headaches.
    5. Padaghata: Located on the soles of the feet. Massaging this area is believed to promote overall relaxation and balance.

Organ reset in ayurveda as well as in functional medicine

In Chinese medicine, emotions are believed to be stored in different organs and their corresponding meridians. For example, anger is associated with the liver, fear with the kidneys, and joy with the heart. The muscles and fascia can also be affected by emotional imbalances, leading to tension and discomfort.

it is believed that the back muscles can store emotions such as stress, tension, and unresolved emotions. Research suggests that poor posture and muscle imbalances can contribute to emotional and psychological stress. By improving posture and addressing any postural defects, it may help alleviate some of the emotional and physical tension stored in the back muscles. It's always beneficial to maintain good posture . Suppressed anger can have a significant impact on the body. When anger is not expressed or dealt with, it can manifest as muscle tension, especially in the back, shoulders, and neck. This tension can lead to chronic pain, headaches, and even digestive issues. It's important to find healthy ways to express and manage anger to maintain overall well-being.

- Multitasking can have a negative impact on women's health, including their organs. When we multitask, our brain has to constantly switch between different tasks, which can lead to increased stress levels and mental fatigue. This can affect the functioning of various organs, such as the brain, heart, and digestive system. It's important to practice self-care and prioritize tasks to minimize the negative effects of multitasking. Liver reset

- Eating light food or avoiding junk food for atleast 7 days help liver to detox itself

Liver reset help increase energy, make you feel calm

In Ayurveda, suppressed anger can affect liver immunity. When anger is not expressed or resolved, it can lead to imbalances in the liver, compromising its function and weakening the immune system. It's important to find healthy ways to manage and release anger to support liver health and maintain a strong immune system. Liver problems have become quite common nowadays. Our liver plays a crucial role in detoxification metabolism, and digestion. With the rise in unhealthy diets, sedentary lifestyles, and exposure to environmental toxins, the liver can face challenges in maintaining optimal function.

Factors like excessive alcohol consumption, poor diet, obesity, viral infections (like Hepatitis), and certain medications can all contribute to liver issues. It's essential to take care of our liver by adopting healthy habits.

Some tips for maintaining a healthy liver include:

In ayurveda or as per recent research Fresh sugarcane juice can indeed be beneficial for liver health! It is believed to have detoxifying properties, liver protective in nature and may help in improving liver function. Sugarcane juice is rich in antioxidants, vitamins, and minerals, which can support liver health and promote its natural detoxification process.

When consuming sugarcane juice for liver health, it's important to keep in mind:Opt for freshly extracted juice: Freshly squeezed sugarcane juice is the best option as it retains the maximum nutrients and enzymes.Overall, incorporating fresh sugarcane juice as part of a balanced and healthy diet can be a refreshing way to support liver health.

- Eating a balanced diet rich in fruits, vegetables, whole grains, and lean proteins.
- Limiting alcohol intake or avoiding it altogether.
- Staying hydrated by drinking enough water throughout the day.
- Engaging in regular exercise to support overall health and weight management.
- Avoiding exposure to toxins and chemicals as much as possible.
- Managing stress levels through relaxation techniques like meditation or yoga.

In Ayurveda, the liver is considered the seat of Pitta dosha, which is responsible for digestion, metabolism, and transformation in the body. When we suppress emotions like anger, it can disturb the balance of Pitta dosha, leading to its accumulation in the liver.

Over time, this accumulation of Pitta dosha in the liver can affect liver function and contribute to issues such as inflammation, impaired detoxification, and even liver disorders.

To maintain a healthy liver and prevent the negative effects of suppressed anger, Ayurveda recommends finding healthy ways to express and manage emotions. This can include practices like mindfulness, meditation, yoga, and engaging in activities that help release emotions in a constructive manner.

Liver function can indeed be related to PCOS (Polycystic Ovary Syndrome). In PCOS, there can be alterations in liver function due to the hormonal imbalances and metabolic disturbances associated with the condition. These alterations may include elevated liver enzymes, such as alanine transaminase (ALT) and aspartate transaminase (AST), indicating liver inflammation or damage.

Walnuts and flaxseeds can be beneficial for liver health! They are both rich in omega-3 fatty acids, antioxidants, and other nutrients that support liver function and promote overall well-being. Omega-3 fatty acids have antiinflammatory properties, which can help reduce inflammation in the liver and support its health. Additionally, the antioxidants found in walnuts and flaxseeds can help protect the liver from oxidative stress and damage.

Including a handful of walnuts or adding flaxseeds to your diet can be a great way to support liver health. You can sprinkle flaxseeds on salads, yogurt, or blend them into smoothies. Walnuts can be enjoyed as a snack

The liver plays a crucial role in hormone metabolism and detoxification. In PCOS, insulin resistance and hormonal imbalances can affect liver function, leading to increased production of androgens (male hormones) and decreased clearance of estrogen from the body. This can contribute to the development and progression of PCOS symptoms.

Maintaining a healthy liver function is important in managing PCOS. This can be achieved through lifestyle modifications such as maintaining a balanced diet, regular exercise, managing body weight, and avoiding excessive alcohol consumption. Additionally, certain Ayurvedic herbs and liver-supportive practices, like consuming bitter foods and herbs, can help support liver health.

It's important to note that individual experiences with PCOS and liver function can vary

- Drinking carrot juice with pinch of black Salt help detox liver

According to recent studies, incorporating carrot juice into your diet can be beneficial for liver health. Carrots are rich in antioxidants and nutrients that support liver function and help protect against liver damage Carrots are a nutritious vegetable that offer several benefits. They are rich in beta-carotene, which is converted into vitamin A in the body. Vitamin A is essential for good vision, healthy skin, and a strong immune system. Carrots are also a good source of fiber, which aids in digestion, and they contain antioxidants that help protect against cell damage. Additionally, carrots provide vitamins C and K, as well as potassium. Including carrots in your diet can help promote overall health and wellbeing. However, it's important to note that carrot juice alone may not be sufficient to maintain liver health. A balanced diet, regular exercise, and avoiding excessive alcohol consumption are also important for overall liver health.

- To reset and support liver health, you can consider incorporating these tips:

1. Increase your intake of liver-friendly foods like leafy greens, beets, garlic, and turmeric.

2. Stay hydrated by drinking plenty of water throughout the day.
3. Limit your alcohol consumption or avoid it altogether.
4. Reduce your intake of processed foods, sugary drinks, and fried foods.
5. Get regular exercise to support overall liver function.
6. Prioritize quality sleep to allow your body to repair and regenerate.
7. Consider incorporating liver-supportive herbs like milk thistle or dandelion root.

- warm water with turmeric is believed to have potential benefits for liver health. Turmeric contains a compound called curcumin, which has antioxidant and anti-inflammatory properties that may support liver function. Adding a pinch of turmeric to warm water and drinking it regularly helps, Curcumin, the active compound in turmeric, has been studied for its potential benefits in improving liver health. It has antioxidant and anti-inflammatory properties that may help protect the liver from damage caused by oxidative stress and inflammation. Additionally, curcumin may support liver function by promoting the production of enzymes that aid in detoxification and by reducing the accumulation of fat in the liver.

- According to recent research Vitamin E can help in reducing non-alcoholic fatty liver and lowering SGPT levels. Vitamin E is an antioxidant that can help protect the liver from damage caused by inflammation and oxidative stress. Non-alcoholic fatty liver disease (NAFLD) is characterized by the accumulation of fat in the liver, which can lead to liver inflammation and elevated SGPT levels. Vitamin E has been studied for its potential in reducing liver inflammation and improving liver function in individuals with NAFLD. It may also help lower SGPT levels, which is a marke' of liver damage. However, it's important to note that the use of Vitamin E for liver health.

Simple breathing technique along with marma or acupressure stimulation to reset your liver and gallbladder

In Ayurveda, the liver marma point is believed to be located in the upper abdomen, just below the right rib cage. It is said to be associated with detoxification and digestion. Stimulating this point may help support liver health and function.

1. Take your right hand's fingure put it on Xyphoid process_
2. go down the rib cage to the right side reach under the rib and push up take your left hand put it behind your neck/trap
3. 3._ breath here 3 time really deep along with pushing that under rib area(breath in here with your mouth means inhale or exhale alternatively with your mouth)
4. now breath in 3 times with your nose inhale or exhale alternatively with your nose

Nowadays toxins or stress accumulation in liver, adrenal gland, kidney causes under eye dark circles, rashes because all these organs need to get relaxed through streching/liver reset breathing technique, psoas release, ileocecal Valve realise, belly button untorque

Belly button untorque

1. To untwist or "untorque" the belly button, you can try gently massaging the area around your belly button in a circular motion. This can help relax any tension or tightness in the muscles and tissues.
2. Put vaccum cupping pump and create vaccum on navel for atleast 10minutes
3. After 10min rolled a cloth put it in chilled water and then put that cloth on navel For sometime, Applying a wet pack to the navel can be a beneficial practice for certain conditions. It is believed to have a cooling and soothing effect on the body, helping to alleviate discomfort and reduce inflammation,

Wet packs work by providing a moist and cooling sensation to the body. When applied to the skin, the moisture from the wet pack evaporates, creating a cooling effect. This can help to reduce heat, soothe inflammation, and provide relief. The wet pack can also help to hydrate the skin and promote relaxation.

Psoas release

The psoas muscle is located deep within the abdomen, connecting the lumbar spine to the femur (thigh bone). It runs from the lower back, passes through the pelvis, and attaches to the top of the thigh bone. Its location makes it an important muscle for hip flexion and stability.

Psoas release techniques can help alleviate tension and tightness in the psoas muscle, promoting relaxation and flexibility. Stretching, massage, and specific exercises are commonly used for psoas release.

• When the psoas muscle is tight, it can cause various symptoms such as lower back pain, hip pain, limited hip mobility, pelvic floor dysfunction, and even digestive issues. It's important to address tightness in the psoas muscle to prevent these symptoms and promote overall flexibility and well-being.

1. How to release your psoas muscle this is the deepest muscle in your core and it's very difficult to release
2. All you need is to rolled a towel, have the towel horizontal on floor
3. Our belly button is directly overtop of the towel this will be painful as you settle in
4. So let's connect to the breath as you inhale expand the belly into the towel
5. As you exhale make the belly nice and small.
6. And when you exhale that's when you start feeling more pain surfacing
7. You can spend minimum 3 minutes here the longer you spend the more benefit you will get.
8. When you are ready place your hand under the shoulder exhale up and off

Benefits of psoas release

Psoas muscle is the only muscle in the body that connects your upper and lower body together and it's very important to release which will help

significantly with back pain

Supplement like Irish sea moss (enriched with minerals), diatomaceous earth supplements help

Sometimes reason of rashes and acne is due to disturbed digestive enzymes in stomach like low levels of proteolytic enzymes can cause disturb digestion results in ache, rashe many more diesease so including papaya, avocado, pineapple rich in proteolytic enzymes helps in improving digestion and reduce acne rashes.

Low levels of proteolytic enzymes can also cause joint pain Because low levels of digestive enzymes causes impaired digestion inturn increase toxins byproduct and get accumulated in joints, Symptoms of low levels of proteolytic enzymes can include difficulty digesting protein-rich foods, bloating, gas, indigestion, and nutrient deficiencies.

Adequate levels of proteolytic enzymes are essential for proper digestion and nutrient absorption.

Supplement of vitamin B6/pyridoxine helps in proper metabolism and overall digestion, Vitamin B6 plays a crucial role in metabolism by helping convert food into energy. It is involved in the metabolism of carbohydrates, proteins, and fats, and also plays a role in the synthesis of neurotransmitters and red blood cells. Adequate levels of vitamin B6 are important for maintaining a healthy metabolism and overall energy production in the body. hence reduces symptoms of skin issues, acne or undereye dark circles

In Ayurveda Nabhi puran/belly button massage is also recommended in such issues

Important marma points or Acupressure points in liver diesease

Marma points are specific points on the body that are vital energy centers in Ayurveda. They are said to be located at the intersections of muscles, bones, joints, tendons, and nerves.

Stimulating these points through massage or pressure is thought to promote balance and healing in the body.

Pressing minimum 9 times at the given specific point causes instant relief

- Hand and leg indravasti marma_ indravasti marma located at centre of Arm, in leg located at centre of calf
- Ani_ Lower region of upper arm
- Urvi_ located at mid region of upper thigh, "Urvi Marma" in Ayurveda refers to an important point in the body. It is located in the middle part of the foot and is considered as a vital energy point. Maintaining the balance of this Marma can improve overall health and well-being.
- manibandh_ at junction of forearm and hand, Manibandh Marma is another important marma point in Ayurveda. It is located around the wrist area. Stimulating this marma point can help with various health issue, Manibandh Marma has several benefits. It can help improve blood circulation in the arms and hands, relieve pain and stiffness, and promote overall wellness in that area. Stimulating this marma point can also have a calming effect on the mind and help reduce stress.
- Stanrohit_ above nipples (pectoralis major),
- Stanmool_ at the base of breast
- Ansphalak_ located at upper back on either side of vertebral column
- Gulph _ at junction of foot and leg(ankle joint) **Bile organ**

Cholesterol precursors, such as cholesterol esters and cholesterol sulfate, are converted into primary bile acids in the liver. These primary bile acids, like cholic acid and chenodeoxycholic acid, are then conjugated with the amino acids glycine or taurine to form bile salts. Bile salts are essential for the emulsification and absorption of dietary fats. They help break down fats into smaller droplets, increasing their surface area for efficient digestion by enzymes. Ultimately, the synthesis and conversion of cholesterol precursors into bile acids are vital for the formation and function of bile in the body.

- Improper bile function can disrupt the body's natural detoxification process, leading to a buildup of toxins in the body. These toxins can affect the health of the skin, leading to increased sebum production and clogged pores. This can result in the formation of comedones, such as blackheads and whiteheads. Restoring proper bile function and supporting the body's detoxification processes can help improve skin health and reduce the occurrence of comedones.
- To correct bile function, it's important to focus on supporting liver health and promoting proper digestion. This can be achieved through dietary changes, such as consuming foods that promote liver function like leafy greens, beets, and dandelion root. Additionally, incorporating bitter herbs like gentian and milk thistle can help stimulate bile production. Regular exercise, staying hydrated, and managing stress levels can also contribute to optimal bile function.
- In Parpati Kalpana, the use of a banana leaf is believed to enhance the production of bile juice. The banana leaf

has properties that promote this increase in bile secretion. This is because the banana leaf is considered kashaya in nature, which means it has an astringent taste and can have beneficial effects on digestion.

- The increased bile juice production can aid in digestion and help regulate the digestive process. It's interesting how Ayurveda incorporates different natural elements like banana leaves to create unique preparations like Parpati Kalpana.The chemical composition of Parpati Kalpana includes HgS (mercury sulfide), which is used in the treatment of digestive disorders. HgS helps improve the functioning of the digestive system and regulates metabolism.That's intresting! Parpati Kalpana,, involves using a banana leaf which enhances the binding power of chlorophyll oxygen. This, in turn, increases the bile juice inside the leaf. The banana leaf is kashaya in nature, meaning it has an astringent taste, and Parpati Kalpana is known to be used in conditions like diarrhea (Atisar) due to its yogvahi nature, which means it helps in absorbing excess liquid.Parpati Kalpana holds great importance in Ayurveda for its role in promoting healthy bile function and treating bilerelated diseases. The unique formulations of Parpati Kalpana help regulate the secretion and flow of bile, which is essential for digestion and maintaining overall digestive health.
- By enhancing bile function, Parpati Kalpana aids in the proper breakdown and absorption of fats, improves metabolism, and supports the elimination of toxins from the body. It is particularly beneficial in conditions like jaundice, gallstones, and other disorders associated with impaired bile production or flow.

- The specific ingredients used in Parpati Kalpana formulations are carefully selected to balance the doshas and restore the optimal functioning of the digestive system. Ayurveda recognizes the significance of bile in maintaining overall wellbeing, and Parpati Kalpana plays a valuable role in supporting healthy bile function.
- When it comes to bloating, bile function is important. Bile helps in the digestion and absorption of fats in the small intestine. If there are issues with bile flow or bile production, it can lead to bloating and digestive discomfort. Maintaining a healthy diet and lifestyle can help support proper bile function and reduce bloating.In Ayurveda, there are several methods to support healthy bile function and reduce bloating. Recommendations include consuming warming spices like ginger and turmeric, incorporating bitter vegetables like bitter gourd and dandelion greens in your diet, practicing stress management techniques like yoga and meditation, and maintaining a regular eating schedule.
- Mixing cumin with lemonade can be a refreshing and natural way to help release gas. Cumin has carminative properties that can aid in digestion and reduce bloating. Try adding a pinch of cumin powder to your lemonade for a flavorful twist that might help ease gas and discomfort. Geera, or cumin powder, is known for its potential to alleviate gas and bloating. It has carminative properties that help reduce gas formation in the digestive tract. You can try adding a pinch of geera powder to your meals or drinking a cup of geera tea to help relieve these symptoms. Universal truth about organic food

- Food or vegetables which is grown root or Tuber of any veggies or fruits and nuts is good for our lower part of body (below navel).
- Like seeds are recommended for reproductive organs Like sesame seeds in amennorhea, Recent studies have shown that sesame seeds can be used as a natural remedy for amenorrhea. Sesame seeds are rich In lignans, which have phytoestrogenic properties that can help regulate hormonal imbalances and promote menstrual regularity. One popular remedy is to consume a teaspoon of roasted sesame seeds with warm water daily.
- sunflower seeds important for male and female fertility enriched with potent fertility nutrients like selenium, zinc, folate. (Cycle 15_28 days/luteal phase),

Sunflower seeds are often included in the second phase of the cycle, known as the luteal phase. They are rich in vitamin E, zinc, and healthy fats, which can help support progesterone production and promote hormonal health. Incorporating sunflower seeds into your diet during the appropriate phase of the cycle may help regulate your menstrual cycle and support overall hormonal balance.

- Flax seeds favour ovulation increase estrogen, In Ayurveda, flax seeds, also known as Alsi, are highly regarded for their medicinal properties. They are considered to be a rich source of essential fatty acids, particularly omega-3 fatty acids, which are beneficial for heart health and reducing inflammation in the body. Flax seeds are also known for their high fiber content, which can aid in digestion and promote healthy bowel movements. In Ayurveda, flax seeds are often recommended for their cooling properties and are used to balance excess heat in the body.

and pumpkin seeds also known as pepitas it is rich source of magnesium help (cycle 1_14 days/follicular phase)also balance hormones during menstruation cycle and help relieve migraine or pain

Ayurvedic tounge analysis(Sensory organ analysis)

Ayurvedic tongue analysis is a practice where the appearance of the tongue is observed to gain insights into one's overall health and imbalances. In Ayurveda, the tongue is considered a reflection of the doshas and their balance in the body. By examining the color, coating, shape, and other characteristics of the tongue, an Ayurvedic practitioner can assess any underlying imbalances and recommend specific dietary and lifestyle changes to restore balances

Vata imbalance _ cracked and dry toungue other symptoms are anxiety, depression, constipation

- Pitta imbalance _ imflammed toungue sometimes with blisters
- Kapha imbalance _ white coated toungue Other symptoms are heavyness in body
- According to Kriya Kala, tongue analysis is believed to provide insights into the progression of diseases. Changes in the color, texture, coating, or markings on the tongue are thought to reflect imbalances in the body. It's an interesting concept, like

1. tip of toungue shows condition of brain health
2. Above tip neck

Herbs or preparation which balances tridosha (body humor)

- Basic way to balance our tridosha or body humor is
- Wakeing up early which balance kapha dosha, sleeping early morning can aggrevate kapha dosha
- Eating light food or easily digestible food help balance pitta dosha
- Avoid staying late night or sleeping early at night help vata dosha balance
- To balance the body humor, Ayurveda suggests following a balanced diet, incorporating herbs and spices that support digestion, and practicing stress management techniques such as meditation or yoga. It is also important to maintain a healthy lifestyle and listen to your body's needs.

Panchamrit best preparation to balance tridosha especially use in rainy season(tridosha imbalance)where imbalances in body due to change in season

. ingredients of panchamrit are milk, curd, honey, ghee, Mishri (rock candy)mix all five and drink Note – honey and ghee unequal quantity

Amla/ emblica officinalis_ also balance tridosha

Emblica officinalis, also known as Amla or Indian Gooseberry, is considered a tridosha ghan in Ayurveda. This means that it has balancing effects on all three doshas – Vata, Pitta, and Kapha. Amla is highly regarded for its numerous health benefits and is often used in Ayurvedic remedies and formulations. It is known for its antioxidant properties, which help in supporting overall wellbeing and boosting the immune system.

Additionally, Amla is believed to promote healthy digestion, enhance hair and skin health, and support the body's natural detoxification processes. It can be consumed in various forms, including fresh fruit, juice, or as supplement.

Basic colour therapy in blood disorder or skin issues

- Wearing green colour cloth is good for vata pitta imbalances
  Green colour is made out from combination of blue and yellow colour
- blue colour especially balance pitta, mostly skin diesease with burn, rashes and redness is caused by pitta imbalances
- Skin diesease with symptoms of scaling or dryness is caused by imbalance of vata so yellow colour cloth is recommended but mostly skin issues is caused by both vata and pitta imbalances so wearing green cloth is better
- Drinking water in sun charged green bottle is good for blood disorder or skin issues, moon charged water is also good and shooting in nature.
- Eating green vegetables is also recommended but warm green vegetables like bitter gourd should be avoided in warm season
- Taking vitamin D is also important but in pitta imbalances directly sunlight on chest should be avoided

can aggrevate pitta and back sun exposure is good in this situation

Neck

Back of the neck hold fear

Miracle remedies using common herbs

Wonder herbs or remedies in ayurveda or multipurpose utilities, tried and tested result Hingu _ very common herb in Indian kitchen

Hingu (Ferula asafoetida)_ very common herb in Indian kitchen is hingu and very potent in many diesease, works wonder in malaria patientsfor prevention

Malaria _

Malaria _ in malaria use as a prophylaxis, fried hingu in ghee(clarified butter) Consume it and put it in clothes use as sniffing

CBD stone (common bile duct stone)_ hingu and takr (buttermilk) lep or application on abdomen can expels out partilom vayu means correct vitiated vata dosha and help in breakdown or exples stone and can prevent surgery.

- Hingwadi kwath can be beneficial in relieving hiccups (hikka) as it helps to improve digestion and reduce gas. It is believed to have a soothing effect on the digestive system, which can help alleviate hiccups.
- Ghee fried hingu (asafoetida) with warm water or ghee fried hingu with buttermilk or ghee fried hingu with with haritki black salt mix with any of buttermilk or warm water can be beneficial in condition of inflammatory bowel syndrome (IBS) for digestion assosiated with vata kapha grahni or IBS and ama mala . It may help with bloating and discomfort.

Note _ Examination of Ama mala in ayurveda is if feces float over water it's is normal mala or feces if feces sit down water means it's Ama mala and we need to incorporate pachana ausadhi.

The powder of Ghee fried hing, marich, pippli, sonth, sendha namak, and vidang, when licked with honey or ghee, is believed to have properties that can help with kasa (cough), dyspnea (difficulty breathing), hiccups, and other respiratory issues. These ingredients are known for their antimicrobial, expectorant, and bronchodilator properties, which may help alleviate symptoms. However, it's important to consult with an Ayurvedic practitioner for personalized guidance and to ensure this remedy is suitable for your specific condition.

- Consumption of pure hingu with ghee Help alivate makkal sula/peuperal after pain, After giving birth, many women experience postpartum after pains. These pains are caused by the retained blood in umbilical area, bladder, hypogastric region caused by vitiated vayu or vata dosha due to this there is severe needle pricking pain in lower abdomen, flatulence or retention of urine also present, In Ayurveda, there are various remedies that can help alleviate these after pains, such as warm herbal teas, gentle abdominal massages with warm oils, and practicing relaxation techniques like deep breathing.

Note_ Hingu, or asafoetida, should be avoided in Raktagulma (blood disorders) because it is believed to aggravate Pitta dosha, which can worsen the condition.

Raktgulm involves an imbalance in Pitta dosha, leading to vitiation of the blood. This vitiated blood can

accumulate in various tissues and organs, causing symptoms associated with blood disorders. The abhisyandi nature of certain foods, including curd, is believed to contribute to the pathogenesis of Raktgulm by creating excess mucus and obstructing the channels through which blood flows.

In Ayurveda, Raktgulm in women refers to blood disorders specific to the female reproductive system. It can manifest as irregular menstrual cycles, heavy bleeding, painful periods, and other related symptoms. Balancing Pitta dosha help manage this condition.

Triphala, mulethi

In market nowadays there are very popular formulations of triphala are like triphala shampoo, triphala eyewash, triphala tablet, triphala churna

Triphala is an herbal remedy used in Ayurveda that consists of three fruits: Amalaki (Indian gooseberry), Bibhitaki, and Haritaki. It is known for its various health benefits and is commonly used to support digestion, promote detoxification, and enhance overall well-being. Triphala is believed to have a balancing effect on the three doshas (Vata, Pitta, and Kapha) and can help improve digestion, regulate bowel movements, and support healthy skin. It can be taken in powder or capsule form and is typically consumed before bed or in the morning on an empty stomach.

I personally tried triphala powder for my scalp dandruff, scalping and hairfall

- Just boil triphala powder and cool it down wash your head or scalp,
  It doesn't show immediate result but hairfall stops immediately if we use frequently.
  Triphala is known to have benefits for the skin. It is believed to help improve skin complexion, reduce inflammation, and promote healthy skin. Its antioxidant properties can help protect the skin from damage caused by free radicals. Triphala can be used topically as a face mask or mixed with water to create a paste.
- Triphala eye wash same boil triphala powder and cool it down and wash your eyes especially in eye redness or eye flu it helps
- Triphala tablet or churna in bloating helps

Marich (piper nigrum)

- Marich (black pepper) is considered to have parmathi (hot) property in Ayurveda, which means it has a cleansing effect on the srotas (channels) in the body. It helps to clear any blockages or stagnation in the channels, promoting better flow of energy and nutrients throughout the body. This cleansing property of marich can help improve digestion, remove toxins, and support overall health. Chedan property in marich refers to the ability of certain substances to penetrate or permeate tissues and cells. It is associated with the sharp and piercing qualities of herbs and their ability to break down blockages, remove toxins, and promote the flow of energy and fluids in the body.

In Ayurveda, wet (snigdha) and dry (ruksha) are two qualities used to describe substances, including herbs like Marich (black pepper). Wet Marich is often used in Ayurvedic remedies that require a milder and nourishing effect, such as soothing digestive teas or herbal tonics. Dry Marich, on the other hand, is commonly used in remedies that aim for a more stimulating and invigorating effect, like respiratory blends or detoxifying formulations. It's important to consider the desired qualities and effects when choosing between wet and dry Marich for Ayurvedic remedies.

- Kshay kasa can occur due to vitiated agni (digestive fire) and imbalance of the three doshas (vata, pitta, and kapha). Kshay kasa, in Ayurveda, refers to a type of cough known as "consumptive cough" or "wasting cough." It is characterized by a persistent cough that leads to weakness, weight loss, and fatigueDurgandit (foul smell) and Kaf (phlegm) are often associated with Kshay Kasa (chronic cough). Marich ghee, honey, and sugar are recommended for kshay kasa. They can help provide strength and aid in reducing the cough.
- Trikatu is a popular Ayurvedic formulation made up of three spices: ginger, black pepper, and long pepper. It is commonly used to support digestion, improve metabolism, and alleviate respiratory congestion. Trikatu is known for its warming and stimulating properties.

Yes, in Ayurveda, Trikatu mixed with buttermilk can be used to help with conditions like Jalodar (ascites). It is believed to improve digestion, reduce bloating, and alleviate fluid retention in the abdomen.

Mulethi

- I personally use mulethi paste in any kind of burn or blisters in mouth (mouth ulcer), just make paste out of mulethi powder and apply it because of it's antiinflammatory or shooting effect it give instant relief.
- Preparing mulethi manth can be a safe and effective option in dehydration. To make mulethi tea, boil mulethi root in water and then add mishri. It can help replenish your body with essential fluids and natural elements. Remember to drink water regularly to combat dehydration.
- Mulethi and madhu (honey) they can be used together for their potential health benefits. Mulethi, also known as licorice root, is often used in Ayurveda for its soothing properties. When combined with madhu(honey), it can create a natural remedy that may help soothe the throat and alleviate coughing or hiccups
- Mulithi (Licorice) is commonly used as an adjuvant in oleation therapy in Ayurveda. When it comes to skin care, some tips include using licorice-infused products for its soothing and brightening properties, applying a paste made from licorice powder and rose water for a healthy glow, and drinking licorice tea to promote overall skin health. Keep your skin happy and glowing That's a great combination for skincare! Mulethi (licorice) and ghee (clarified butter) can be mixed together to make a nourishing face mask. Olive oil is also fantastic for skin hydration. Give it a try and enjoy the benefits of these natural ingredients for your skin!

- Mulethi, also known as licorice root, is a popular herb in Ayurveda with various medicinal properties. It is used in Ayurvedic remedies for a wide range of health concerns. Mulethi is believed to have antiinflammatory, antioxidant, and antimicrobial properties Mulethi has a sweet taste (ras), a cooling effect (guna), and a sweet post-digestive effect (vipaka) in Ayurveda.. It can be beneficial for respiratory health, soothing coughs and sore throats. Mulethi is also used to support digestive health, promote liver function, and balance hormones, The usable part of Mulethi, also known as Licorice, is the root and root extract. It is commonly used in various forms like powder, tea, or as an ingredient in herbal remedies. Mulethi is known for its sweet taste and medicinal properties, which can help with digestive issues, cough, sore throat, and other ailments.
- In the context of Ayurveda, a mixture of Mulethi, Black clay, sankh, rice water and honey can be used in the treatment of bloody diarrhea modern medical terminology, "bloody diarrhea" is commonly referred to as "hematochezia." Rice water can help improve digestion, while honey can provide soothing effects to the stomach, mulethi protect mucous layer of gastrointestinal tract
- Mulethi with ghee can be used in a cold tampon for threatened abortion or to provide relief in pregnancy complications.
- Mulethi churna can be used for massaging on kikkisa or striae gravidarum to help reduce their appearance.

- Khadir (Acacia catechu) is act as a blood purifier in pigmentation or skin issues, khadir powder boiled and cool it down and drink sip by sip .
- Khadir contains various chemical constituents that contribute to its medicinal properties. Some of the key constituents found in Khadir include catechins, flavonoids, tannins, alkaloids, and phenolic compounds. These compounds are responsible for the antimicrobial, anti-inflammatory, and antioxidant effects of Khadir, The usable part of Khadir, which is also known as Acacia catechu, is the bark and roots. It is commonly used in various skincare products and remedies due to its antimicrobial, antifungal, and anti-inflammatory properties. The bark and root extracts of Khadir are used in powders, oils, or skincare products.
- Tandulodak, or rice water, is a traditional remedy used in Ayurveda for various purposes. It is believed to have cooling and soothing properties, making it beneficial for conditions like indigestion, diarrhea, and skin irritations. To prepare tandulodak, simply rinse rice and collect the water that remains after the rice has been soaked or cooked. This water can be consumed as a drink or used topically on the skin.Tandulodak, or rice water, can be used as a remedy for leucorrhoea in Ayurveda. It is believed to have cooling and cleansing properties that can help alleviate the symptoms of leucorrhoea. To use tandulodak for this condition, you can consume it as a drink or use it as a vaginal wash.
- Tandulodak, or rice water, can be used as a remedy for vomiting in Ayurveda. It is believed to have a calming effect on the stomach and can help soothe the digestive

system. To use tandulodak for vomiting, you can consume small sips of rice water mix with chaturjaat or sarkara for better taste throughout the day.

- In the context of Ayurveda, a mixture of rice water and honey can be used in the treatment of bloody diarrhea In modern medical terminology, "bloody diarrhea" is commonly referred to as

"hematochezia." . Rice water can help improve digestion, while honey can provide soothing effects to the stomach. Coriander

- Dhaniya (coriander) belongs to the Harit Varga (taken in raw form or green category) in Ayurveda. It is considered tridosha-nashak, meaning it helps balance all three doshas.
- soaking coriander seeds in water overnight strain it and mix honey in it and drinking the water in the morning is believed to have various health benefits. It can help improve digestion, reduce inflammation, help alivate excess thrist and detoxify the body. In Ayurveda, soaking coriander seeds in water is believed to have a cooling effect on the body. It can help balance excess heat and reduce Pitta dosha. Give it a try for a refreshing and cooling effect
- Coriander is believed to have diuretic properties, which means it may help promote kidney health and improve urine flow. It is commonly used in Ayurveda for its detoxifying and cleansing effects on the kidneys.Boiling coriander leaves for kidney health is not a common practice in Ayurveda. However, coriander leaves have cooling properties and are rich in antioxidants. They may

support overall kidney health by promoting detoxification and reducing inflammation.

- In Ayurveda, dhaniya (coriander) is considered an important herb with various health benefits. It is believed to have a cooling effect on the body, aiding in digestion and reducing inflammation. Dhaniya is also rich in antioxidants and essential nutrients like vitamins A, C, and K. It can be used in various forms like fresh leaves, dried seeds, or as a spice in cooking. Incorporating dhaniya into your diet can promote overall well-being.
- In Ayurveda, dhaniya (coriander) can be beneficial after a prolonged delivery or dukhparsav. It is believed to have properties that help in postpartum healing and recovery. Dhaniya can help with digestion, reduce inflammation, and provide essential nutrients. It can be consumed as a tea, added to meals, or used in herbal remedies.
- In Ayurveda, dhaniya (coriander) is believed to have properties that can help with pandu (anemia). It is considered to be rich in iron, which is essential for the production of healthy red blood cells. Consuming dhaniya regularly can help improve hemoglobin levels and combat anemia. It can be added to meals, juices, or taken in the form of dhaniya water for its beneficial effects.
- pomegranate can be garnished with coriander leaves to enhance the flavor and add a nutritional boost. However, for specifically boosting iron levels, consuming pomegranate and coriander together good for Anemic patients.
- To make dhaniya leaf boiled water, follow these steps:

1. Take a handful of fresh dhaniya leaves.

2. Wash the leaves thoroughly to remove any dirt or impurities.
3. Boil a cup of water in a pot.
4. Add the washed dhaniya leaves to the boiling water.
5. Let it simmer for about 5-10 minutes.
6. Turn off the heat and strain the dhaniya leaves from the water.
7. Allow the boiled water to cool down.
8. You can drink this dhaniya leaf boiled water as it is or add a squeeze of lemon for extra flavor.

Remember, this is a traditional remedy, and individual results may vary.

To combat anemia, you can try these remedies using dhaniya (coriander):

1. Dhaniya Juice: Blend fresh dhaniya leaves with water to make a juice. Drink this juice regularly to boost iron levels and combat anemia.
2. Dhaniya Salad: Include fresh dhaniya leaves in your salads. Its iron content can help in the production of red blood cells and improve hemoglobin levels.
3. Dhaniya Infusion: Boil dhaniya seeds in water and strain the infusion. Drink this concoction regularly to increase iron absorption and alleviate anemia symptoms.

   To harness the benefits of dhaniya (coriander), you can try these remedies:

4. Dhaniya Water: Soak a handful of dhaniya seeds in water overnight. Drink the infused water in the morning to aid digestion and detoxify the body.

5. Dhaniya Tea: Boil crushed dhaniya seeds in water for a few minutes. Strain and drink the tea to soothe digestive issues and promote overall well-being.
6. Dhaniya Paste: Make a paste by grinding fresh dhaniya leaves and apply it to skin irritations or insect bites for relief.

Munnaka

- Munnaka, or raisins, are considered to have a mridu virechana (gentle purgative) effect in Ayurveda. This means that they can help promote healthy bowel movements and relieve constipation . In Ayurveda, munnaka can be beneficial in ksaya kasa

  (consumptive cough) with excess dosha. It helps in nourishing the body, providing strength, and reducing cough symptoms. Munnaka, also known as raisins, has therapeutic uses in Ayurveda. It is used to enhance digestion, increase weight, provide freshness, and strengthen the body. Regular consumption of munnaka is beneficial for the body.

- During digestion, pittaj gulma can cause intense pain and symptoms similar to varan (obstruction). Eating munnaka can provide relief in such cases.According to Ayurveda, the pathogenesis of gulma involves an imbalance of doshas, particularly vata and kapha, leading to the formation of a mass or obstruction in the abdominal region. In modern medicine, gulma is often referred to as an abdominal mass or tumor. It can be caused by various factors such as hernias, tumors, or cysts. This can cause symptoms such as pain, distension, and digestive disturbances. Treatment aims to balance the doshas and remove the obstruction through various Ayurvedic therapies and lifestyle modifications.

Virechana with munnaka hartki swaras and gud helps relieve pittaj gulma

- Munnaka (raisins) can be helpful in managing pittaj madatya (alcohol intoxication). It is believed that munnaka helps in reducing the effects of alcohol and provides relief from symptoms like nausea and headache.

Erand oil use

Erand oil, also known as castor oil, is commonly used in Ayurveda for its beneficial properties in Vataj Grahni. Grahni means "duodenum agni ashray" in English, which refers to the duodenum being the seat of digestive fire and its role in digesting uncooked food. Its position is above navel, Vataj Grahni refers to a condition characterized by imbalanced Vata dosha in the gastrointestinal tract. Erand oil is believed to help pacify Vata dosha and promote healthy digestion. It has a warming effect on the body and can help alleviate symptoms like abdominal pain, bloating, and irregular bowel movements. However, it's important to consult with an Ayurvedic practitioner before using erand oil

If you're experiencing flatulence and dry feces comes with difficulty and after straining for sometime with toxins in Vataj Grahni, using erand oil (castor oil) may help. It can aid in lubricating the intestines, promoting proper bowel movements, and reducing toxins.

In Vataj Grahni, one may experience an increased desire to eat all tastes (rasa), along with mental distress (mansik avsad), cough and breathlessness (kasa swas), heart disease, abdominal pain (gulm), and spleen-related issues.

- Kaphaavrit vata refers to the vitiation of vata dosha due to the accumulation of kapha dosha. In Ayurveda, the use of erand oil (castor oil) is recommended for balancing kapha and vata doshas. Erand oil has a heating effect and helps to alleviate excess kapha and improve digestion.
- In case pitta or kapha envolved coughing erand oil can be used as sneh virechana or as purgative therapy.
- Erand oil use in anah constipation belching with pinas mainly use as purgative therapy in girdasi, paralysis pakshavad, or in case of vata obstruction by excess kaphameda pitta rakta (medaraktpittakaphasansargajvata nasak)

Quantity in these chronic issues are approx 200 ml it's must to assess condition of patients before use

Anupana or erand oil should be taken with milk, triphala kwath, mugdyush, as per diesease condition

- If you have inflammation and vatasang-related issues, you can use castor oil before meals Along with mansrasa or broth It provides calmness and relief to the body.
- Erand oil can be used in The condition of

Purishavritvata in Ayurveda refers to an imbalance of Vata dosha, which affects the normal functioning of bowel movements. It can lead to irregularity, instability, and inconsistency in the stool. Fast digestion of ghee after meal Ayurveda suggests making changes in diet and lifestyle to restore balance in this condition.Erand oil can be beneficial for belching and intermittent defecation pain in the back, pelvis, sacrum, and for an unhealthy heart.

- Vayanavrit vata, or a condition of disturbed vata in the intestines, can have correlations with PCOS, flatulence, and belching, parikartika, vomiting endometriosis It is important to address the underlying vata imbalance and make dietary and lifestyle changes here erand oil pack for abdomen is beneficial, warm erand oil should be dip in clothes then put it on abdomen for vataanuloman and PCOS reduction.

Haritaki (Terminelia chebula)

- If you have inflammation with diarrhea or dysentery, "gudabhya" refers to using jaggery with haritaki powder or sonth /dry ginger with jaggery powder. It can have beneficial properties for digestion and soothing effects. Consult your Ayurvedic practitioner for proper dosage
- In Ayurveda, Haritaki lep (paste) is believed to be beneficial for reducing acne marks. It is said to have properties that help lighten the appearance of acne scars and promote healthier skin. Haritaki powder is considered beneficial for acne in Ayurveda. It has antimicrobial and antiinflammatory properties that can help reduce acne-causing bacteria and inflammation. You can make a paste using Haritaki powder and mix it with water or other natural ingredients like honey or rose water. Apply the paste to the acne marks and leave it on for some time before rinsing off.Haritaki powder is highly valued in Ayurveda for its properties in treating acne. It possesses antimicrobial and anti-inflammatory properties that help reduce inflammation, fight bacteria,

and unclog pores. It can be used in face masks or as a paste with other natural ingredients to target acne-prone skin and promote a clearer complexion

Note _According to some beliefs in Ayurveda, cow milk is thought to contain hormones that may disrupt the natural balance in the body and contribute to hormonal issues, including acne. Buffalo milk is considered a healthier alternative if someone suffering from acne.

- In Ayurveda, Haritaki (Terminalia chebula) is often used for sodhan (cleansing) in cases of excess dosha, such as in Atisar (diarrhea). Haritaki is believed to have a cleansing effect on the digestive system, helping to balance the doshas and alleviate symptoms of diarrhea. It is recommended to consult with an Ayurvedic practitioner for proper usage and dosage guidance.
- In Ayurveda, Haritaki is commonly used for the management of hemorrhoids. It is believed to have anti-inflammatory and astringent properties that can help reduce swelling and discomfort associated with hemorrhoids. It is recommended to consult with an Ayurvedic practitioner for personalized advice on how to use Haritaki for hemorrhoids.

Structured water/Hydration to avoid diesease

Our cell is made up (structured water)H3o2, structured water inside in our cell prevent diesease, cancer, premature ageing

Lack of structured water inside our cell can leads to incorrect protein folding, diesease and dehydrated cell.

- Structured water is believed to have several potential benefits. According to recent studies, structured water may have improved hydration properties, increased bioavailability of nutrients, and enhanced cellular function. It is also thought to support better digestion, detoxification, and overall well-being. While more research is needed to fully understand the benefits of structured water, incorporating hydration habits that promote its formation, such as consuming fresh fruits and vegetables, may be beneficial for maintaining optimal health.
- In ayurveda or dynamic it's understood as water element helps in tissue binding, without water element or in condition of chronic dehydration tissue will not bind together so healing is not possible
- According to recent studies, structured water can be found in certain natural sources such as flowing rivers, streams, and waterfalls. The movement and exposure to natural electromagnetic fields are believed to enhance the structure of the water molecules .
- fresh fruits and vegetables are considered good sources of structured water. These foods contain high water

content and are believed to have a more organized molecular structure, which can contribute to better hydration and overall health.

Sources of structured water

Minerals and nutrient rich fruits and vegetables

Structured water rich fruits and vegetables are watermelon, cucumber, mushroom, carrot, strawberry, spinach, Bell pepper

- Herb infused water like khas water, To infuse Khas waterDrinking Khas water infusion is a traditional remedy used in Ayurveda to help balance the body's pH levels and promote alkalinity. It involves infusing water with Khas roots (Vetiver roots) to create a refreshing and cooling drink. This remedy is believed to have a calming effect on the body and can be enjoyed throughout the day. you can follow these steps:
    1. Take a handful of Khas roots (Vetiver roots) and wash them thoroughly.
    2. Place the washed Khas roots in a clean container or pitcher.
    3. Pour about 1 liter of water over the Khas roots.
    4. Let the Khas roots soak in the water for at least 46 hours, or overnight for a stronger infusion.
    5. After the infusion period, strain the water to remove the Khas roots.
    6. Your Khas water infusion is now ready to be enjoyed! You can drink it throughout the day to promote alkalinity and a sense of calmness.
- cucumber infused water is good for dehydration,

- Mineral rich water or lemonade with rock salt also good to boost natural energy level

Note_ tomato is rich in structured water upto 95percentage but it's also comes under nightshade, so person suffering with inflammation or any inflammatory diesease should avoid tomato, In Ayurveda, nightshade vegetables like tomatoes are considered to have a heating (pitta-aggravating) effect on the body, which can potentially worsen inflammation.

- According to recent studies, tomatoes and nightshade vegetables contain a compound called solanine, which may trigger inflammation in some individuals. However, it's important to note that the relationship between nightshades and inflammation is not well-established and may vary from person to person.

Different types of water and it's utilities

1. In Ayurveda, the practice of boiling and cooling down water is believed to have potential benefits. It is thought to help balance the doshas, improve digestion, good for inflammatory diesease, diarrhoea, blood disorder, hallucinations, poisoning, excess thrist, vomiting and good in any kind of intoxication or hangover,

   Boiling water is a common method for water purification. It helps kill or inactivate harmful microorganisms, making the water safer to drink.

2. In Ayurveda, drinking cold water is believed to have several benefits. It helps to cool down the body and pacify the pitta dosha. It may also help reduce inflammation and congestion in the respiratory system,

cold water is advisable in unconscious person, pitta or inflammatory diesease, summer season, poisoning, blood disorder, intoxication, fatigue, vomiting, nose bleeding, Asthma/tamak swas if it aggrevate at night time and feel dizzy or caused by pollution, belching, indigestion, vegadharan than cold water is advisable, Tamak swas, or asthma, is a type of chronic respiratory disease in modern science. It is characterized by inflammation and narrowing of the airways. The main causes can include genetic predisposition, allergens, air pollution, and lifestyle factors. In modern medicine, it is treated with bronchodilators, corticosteroids, and lifestyle changes.

Note – Asthma with fever and unconscious cold water is not advisable

Workout and exercise according to Ayurveda and sport medicine

- According to sport medicine if we want to increase muscle mass we should not eat anything 1hours before exercise it increases testosterone levels and help building muscle mass.
- Regular workouts and exercise can help reduce inflammation in the body. Following proper workout rules, such as warming up, using proper form, and gradually increasing intensity, can help minimize the risk of inflammation and injury.
- For example some people are prone to inflammation or inflammatory diesease like psoriasis should exercise moderately or after taking advice from their doctors
- For women follicular phase (1 week after period or menses/before ovulation)is best to workout and gain healthy weight in this phase estrogen and testosterone both are high
- While estrogen does play a role in fat distribution, it's important to note that we cannot selectively control where fat is deposited in the body. Balancing estrogen levels involves maintaining overall hormonal balance through a healthy lifestyle, including regular exercise, a balanced diet, stress management, and adequate sleep. These factors contribute to overall wellbeing and can support a healthy body composition.

- High levels of estrogen hormone or cortisol can contribute to belly fat. Exercising at the right time, such as in the morning or before meals, can help burn calories and reduce belly fat. It's important to combine exercise with a balanced diet for optimal results. Estrogen and cortisol can interact in various ways in the body. Cortisol, often referred to as the stress hormone, is produced by the adrenal glands and helps regulate the body's response to stress. When cortisol levels are elevated due to stress, it can have an impact on estrogen levels. High cortisol levels can interfere with the production, release, and function of estrogen, potentially leading to hormonal imbalances. This can affect various aspects of reproductive health, including the menstrual cycle and fertility. However, the exact mechanisms of this interaction are complex and can vary from person to person. It's important to manage stress levels through relaxation techniques, exercise, and self-care to support hormonal balance.
- FSH, or follicle-stimulating hormone, plays a crucial role in the process of aromatization. Aromatization is the conversion of androgens (male hormones) to estrogen (female hormones) in the granulosa cells (GC) of the ovaries. FSH stimulates the granulosa cells to produce aromatase, an enzyme responsible for this conversion.
- However, excessive FSH levels can lead to an excess conversion of androgens to estrogen. This can result in an imbalance of estrogen in the body, which may have harmful effects. Excess estrogen can contribute to conditions such as estrogen dominance, which can cause symptoms like irregular periods, mood swings, and even increase the risk of certain cancers, excess fat

depositsion, so balancing FSH through relaxation teqnique because it's secreted by brain (hypothalamus) is necessary.

non-communicable metabolic diesease epidemiology

Metabolic diseases are conditions that affect the body's metabolism, which is the process of converting food into energy. They often involve abnormalities in how the body processes nutrients, such as carbohydrates, proteins, and fats. Common metabolic diseases include diabetes, obesity, and metabolic syndrome. These conditions can have various symptoms and complications and may require lifestyle changes, medication, or other treatments to manage.

Thyroid hormone related with hpo axis it's disorder causes metabolic diesease In Ayurveda, hypothyroidism is primarily associated with the vitiation of Kapha and Vata doshas. However, when we specifically look at the dosha involved in the manifestation of hypothyroidism, Udana Vayu is often mentioned.

Udana Vayu is a subtype of Vata dosha responsible for the upward movement in the body, including speech, growth, and expression. When Udana Vayu becomes imbalanced, it can affect the functioning of the thyroid gland, leading to symptoms of hypothyroidism.

Imbalance in Udana Vayu can result in symptoms such as fatigue, weight gain, sluggishness, dry skin, constipation, and difficulty in expressing oneself. Ayurveda aims to balance Udana Vayu through specific dietary and lifestyle modifications, herbal remedies, and practices like pranayama (breathing exercises) and yoga.

to correct it Ameen ucharan or Ameen speech therapy helps, Ameen Therapy is a unique approach that combines speech therapy techniques with a holistic healing perspective. It emphasizes the integration of mind, body, and spirit to address communication challenges. Ameen therapy, also known as "Ameen therapy, " is a holistic approach that utilizes the power of sound and vibration to promote healing and well-being. It is based on the principle of the sacred sound ameen which is considered to be the primordial sound of the universe in some traditions. The therapy involves humming (sound made by producing wordless tone with mouth closed forcing the sound to emerge from nose)the sound of ameen to induce relaxation, balance energy, and enhance spiritual and emotional wellbeing. Ameen therapy can be a soothing and transformative practice for those seeking inner peace and harmony.

Humming sound therapy, also known as "mmm therapy, " is a simple and effective technique that involves making a continuous humming sound. It can help promote relaxation, reduce stress, and improve focus. By vibrating the vocal cords, humming produces calming vibrations that can have a soothing effect on the body and mind. It can be done anytime, anywhere, as a self-care practice to bring about a sense of peace and tranquility. Give it a try and see how humming sound therapy can benefit you!

Diabetes a epidemiology

In the context of Madhumeh (diabetes) in Ayurveda, the vitiations of various doshas are described. According to Ayurveda, the imbalances in Prana Vayu, Udana Vayu, Sadhak Pitta, and Bodhak Kapha can contribute to the development of diabetes.

Prana Vayu, a subtype of Vata dosha, is responsible for the intake and circulation of energy and nutrients. When Prana Vayu gets imbalanced, it can manifest as symptoms like excessive thirst and fatigue.

Udana Vayu, another subtype of Vata dosha, is associated with upward movement, including speech and expression. Imbalance in Udana Vayu can lead to symptoms like difficulty in speaking, breathlessness, and dryness.

Sadhak Pitta, a subtype of Pitta dosha, is responsible for maintaining emotional balance, intelligence, and coordination. When Sadhak Pitta is imbalanced, it can result in symptoms like increased irritability, difficulty in concentration, and emotional instability.

Bodhak Kapha, a subtype of Kapha dosha, is associated with perception, understanding, and cognitive functions. Imbalance in Bodhak Kapha can manifest as symptoms like confusion, mental fog, and difficulty in understanding.By analyzing the tongue in Ayurveda, the condition of Bodhak Kapha can be assessed. Bodhak Kapha governs the perception and understanding of taste. In tongue analysis, if there is an excess of Bodhak Kapha, the tongue may appear coated with a thick, white or yellowish coating. This coating may affect the sense of taste, making it dull or distorted. It's important to note that tongue analysis is just one aspect of Ayurvedic diagnosis, and a comprehensive assessment is necessary for accurate evaluation.

Ayurveda aims to balance these doshas through dietary and lifestyle modifications, herbal remedies, and practices like pranayama (breathing exercises), meditation, and yoga. These approaches help in managing diabetes effectively.

- 3 test are there for diabetes is fasting glucose level, Hba1c, OGTT (oral glucose tolerance test,
- In order to test for diabetes, there are three common tests that are typically performed:
  1. Fasting Plasma Glucose (FPG) Test: This test measures your blood sugar level after fasting for at least 8 hours. A blood sample is taken to determine if your glucose level is within the normal range.
  2. Oral Glucose Tolerance Test (OGTT): This test involves drinking a sugary solution and then having your blood sugar levels measured at specific intervals. It helps determine how well your body processes glucose over time.
  3. Hemoglobin A1c (HbA1c) Test: This test measures your average blood sugar levels over the past 2-3 months. It provides a more long-term view of your blood sugar control.
- Naga bhasma, when used in Ayurveda, is believed to help balance and absorb excess kapha dosha, which is associated with water and constructive energy in the body. It may assist in reducing swelling, inflammation, and other disease-causing secretions.

- Naag bhasma 125mg, silajatu, and milk can help reduce excessive thirst in diabetes. They have cooling properties and balance vikrut kapha dosha or even good in case of diabetic gangrene Naga bhasma pb use to treat tridoshaj kapha vikrut disorder balance emerging or constructive energy in body basically kapha/aapt or water part is used as constructive part of body, Naga bhasma absorb vikrut kapha or supporative secretion or kled or disease causing secretion like swelling or inflammation description
- Eating raw salad vegetables before a meal can help prevent a rapid rise in blood sugar levels. The high fiber content in vegetables slows down the digestion and absorption of carbohydrates from the subsequent meal, resulting in a more gradual release of sugar into the bloodstream. This can help maintain stable blood sugar levels and prevent spikes. So, having a salad as a starter can be a smart choicc.

  Having a bowl of salad or veggies before a meal can support healing from chronic diseases by providing essential nutrients, antioxidants, and fiber. These nutrient-dense foods help nourish the body, support the immune system, and promote overall health. Additionally, the high fiber content can aid in digestion, improve gut health, and assist in managing weight, which is important for many chronic conditions. So, incorporating a bowl of salad or veggies into your meals can be a beneficial step towards healing and wellness…
- Food having Low glycemic index must be included in diet like millets(jawar, bajra), Besan etc

- Besan (chicken pea)has a relatively lower glycemic index compared to other flours, making it a good choice for those seeking low glycemic index foods.
- some of the lowest glycemic index foods include non-starchy vegetables like broccoli, spinach, and kale, as well as legumes like lentils and chickpeas. These foods have a minimal impact on blood sugar levels and can be incorporated into a balanced diet for individuals with diabetes.
- Low glycemic index foods are those that have a minimal impact on blood sugar levels. Examples include non-starchy vegetables, legumes, whole grains, and certain fruits like berries and apples. These foods can help maintain stable blood sugar levels and provide sustained energy.
- According to recent studies, a diabetes diet protocol typically focuses on balancing blood sugar levels and promoting overall health. It often involves consuming a variety of nutrient-dense foods, including whole grains, lean proteins, healthy fats, and plenty of fruits and vegetables.
- Portion control, regular meal timings, and monitoring carbohydrate intake are also important aspects of managing diabetes through diet.

Colour of fruits and vegetables health benefits according to colour of fruits and veggies

- Red colour in fruits and vegetables (tomato, apple) is because of antioxidants called lycopene, Lycopene is very important for heart health because it helps in bringing down bad cholesterol LDL and increase good cholesterol that HDL, it also helps in preventing cancer like bone, prostate and lung cancer and it's best anti-ageing Antioxidant

- Lycopene, found in tomatoes, has antiinflammatory properties that may help reduce inflammation associated with endometriosis
- Red-colored fruits, such as strawberries and cherries, are rich in antioxidants polyphenols that can help support heart health and boost the immune system or also nourish adrenal gland
- red-colored fruits like strawberries, cherries, and raspberries are packed with nutrients and antioxidants. They are known for their high content of vitamin C, which supports immune function and collagen production. These fruits also contain powerful antioxidants like anthocyanins, which have been linked to reducing inflammation and promoting heart health. Including red fruits in your diet can provide a range of health benefits and add vibrant color to your meals.

Yellow colour fruits

- Yellow colour fruits are rich in catalytic enzymes like proteolytic enzymes and support pancrease
- yellow-colored fruits like bananas, lemons, and pineapples are rich in essential vitamins, minerals, and antioxidants. They can provide various health benefits, such as boosting immunity, promoting healthy digestion, and supporting eye health. These fruits are also a great source of dietary fiber and can help maintain healthy blood pressure levels.

- According to recent research, fruit juice can be a convenient way to consume essential vitamins and minerals found in fruits. However, it's important to note that some fruit juices can be high in sugar and lack the fiber content found in whole fruits. It's generally recommended to consume whole fruits whenever possible, as they provide more fiber and have a lower glycemic load. If you choose to drink fruit juice, opt for freshly squeezed or 100% fruit juice without added sugars.

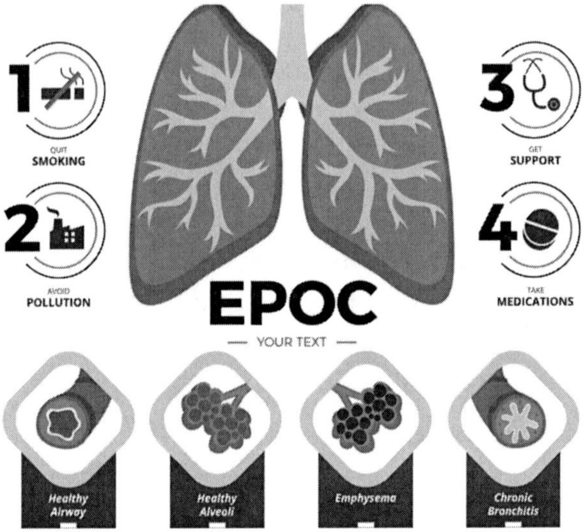

Lungs and it's biophysics and care

Diesease burden in our society and it's control and management

Tuberculosis (TB), malaria, blindness and AIDS all these four diesease was burden in society but nowadays due to National policy and improvement in technology or science somehow reduction in cases of these diesease is seen

1. In present time tuberculosis or other respiratory diesease are Re_emerging diesease

Reemerging means previously controlled by antibiotics or therapy but now they have developed antimicrobial resistance an can be seen as epidemic

B

Biophysics of diesease like tuberculosis, Asthma in Ayurveda and it's prevention

In Asthma or TB initially person is malnourished /weak or in any kind of aptarpanjanya vayadhi means diesease caused by emaciation _ in lungs tissue becomes so weak that causes increase in vata Dosha or after vata aggrevation if person exposes to cold which is same as the property of vata

Due to excessive aggrevation of vata (drying, cooling) lungs start to collapse _ our body try to protect collapsing lung and start building thick mucus plug to protect weak lung tissues _ coughing symptoms start

• Kasa, or coughing, is often considered an initial stage of lung issues. It can be a symptom of various respiratory conditions. Swas, or dyspnea, which refers to difficulty in breathing or shortness of breath, can occur in later stages when the lungs produce mucus to protect their shape. It's important to consult a healthcare professional for a proper diagnosis and treatment.

Prevention is always better than cure _after understating biophysics of respiratory diesease or Asthma some point are clear so that we can prevent these diesease

1. Vegadharan(control over natural urges) should be avoided it also can aggrevate vata dosha
2. disease burden refers to the impact of diseases on a population. It includes factors such as mortality, morbidity, and disability caused by various diseases. Understanding the disease burden helps in prioritizing resources and interventions to reduce the impact of diseases on individuals and communities.
3. In Ayurveda, disease burden is seen as an imbalance in the doshas and the accumulation of toxins in the body. Ayurveda focuses on restoring balance and eliminating toxins through various practices to reduce the burden of diseases and promote overall well-being.
4. After suffering from malnutrition or weakness before recovery cold
5. When it comes to coughing, a traditional Ayurvedic decoction can be made with pippli (long pepper), haldi (turmeric), Kali mirch (black pepper), and adrak (ginger). This decoction is believed to have soothing and expectorant and antibiotics properties.
6. Moon milk is a trendy Ayurvedic preparation that can help promote lung health and aid recovery. To make it, you can prepare a decoction with pippli (long pepper),

haldi (turmeric), Kali mirch (black pepper), sonth (dried ginger), and dates.

Then mix and boil this decoction with warm milk for a soothing and nourishing drink. 🍌🥛 Cheers to healthy lungs!

7. In Ayurveda, Trikatu is a combination of three spices – ginger, black pepper, and long pepper. It is known for its heating and digestive properties. While Trikatu may not directly address sawas or dyspnea, it can help balance vata and pitta doshas, which are often associated with respiratory issues.
8. Vitamin C is important for treating lung tissue because it has antioxidant properties that can help reduce inflammation and oxidative stress in the lungs. It also supports the immune system, which is crucial for maintaining healthy lung function. Including vitamin C-rich foods in your diet or taking supplements can help support lung health.
9. Sitopladi is an Ayurvedic formulation commonly used for respiratory issues like wet cough. It contains ingredients like sugar, vanslochan, pippali, cardamom, and cinnamon. These ingredients are known for their soothing and expectorant properties, which can help relieve cough and congestion, Sitopladi churna is not ruksan means not drying in nature can be beneficial in lungs cancer because in this case dipan pachan brihan required which is achieved by sitopladi description

Ingredients here act especially on pranavah, udan, vah and annvah srotas which is visited in dyspnea or swasa roga

Sitopladi churna is often taken with honey or warm water. It is believed to help with respiratory issues and improve digestion. Anupana refers to the vehicle or medium through which the churna is consumed. In this case, you can mix Sitopladi churna with honey or warm water to consume it.

• Talishadi Churna is an Ayurvedic formulation that typically contains ingredients like talisapatra (Indian bay leaf), pippali (long pepper), ela (cardamom), and sunthi (ginger). It is commonly used for respiratory conditions like cough, cold, and congestion. Talishadi Churna is known for its expectorant and bronchodilator properties, which can help alleviate respiratory symptoms. It is commonly used for dry cough as it has expectorant properties that help in relieving cough and soothing the respiratory tract

10. In Islam, there are some recommended practices for sleeping known as Sunnah. One of the Sunnahs is to sleep on your right side, as it is believed to be the way the Prophet Muhammad (peace be upon him) used to sleep. Additionally, it is encouraged to recite certain supplications before sleeping and to sleep in a state of cleanliness.

11. According to Ayurveda, Sleeping on the right side is believed to increase Kapha dosha according to Ayurveda. However, it is considered a good sleeping position as it can aid digestion and reduce acid reflux.sleeping on your right side is believed to be beneficial for liver health. It helps promote proper digestion and supports the detoxification process of the liver, Sleeping on the right side is considered better than sleeping on the left side because it can help prevent acid reflux by keeping the stomach lower than the esophagus. This position can also aid digestion and promote better blood flow to the heart.

12. According to recent studies, sleeping on your left side is considered beneficial for high blood pressure. It helps improve circulation and reduces the strain on the heart.Sleeping on the left side is believed to increase Pitta dosha in Ayurveda. However, it is considered a good position to sleep because it can promote better digestion and blood circulation. If there any kind of intense pain then left side is recommended, Sleeping on the left side is often recommended for intense pain because it can help relieve pressure on certain organs, such as the liver and stomach. This position can also promote better blood flow and reduce strain on the spine.

Note _In pregnancy, sleeping on the left side is often recommended. This position helps improve blood circulation to the baby and prevents the uterus from pressing on major blood vessels. It can also help reduce swelling and alleviate discomfort.Sleeping on the left side can prevent the uterus from putting pressure on the superior vena cava and the inferior vena cava. This helps improve blood flow to the heart and reduces the risk of complications during pregnancy. It's a recommended position for better circulation.

13. **Reset of lungs or weak tissues within lungs to avoid collapse or mucus plug formation**

Hair care in ayurveda and maintaining all sensory organs

- According to ayurvedic physiology hair is made out of Asthi mala part (excretory part), you can understand byproduct of bones So it's very necessary to takecare of bone health for better hair health
  Asthi bone is made up of 3 mahabhuta which is
- prithvi(prominently form mans muscle tissue),
- Agni mahabhuta (prominently form blood tissue)
- Vayu mahabhuta (which fill space)
- So taking care of all three mahabhuta or muscle health and blood health (circulation) helps better hair improvement.
- Another important ritual in ayurveda for better hair health is Nasya
- Nasya is a major Ayurvedic treatment that can help improve hair health. It delivers medicine into the body through the nose and enhances blood circulation. This can lead to improved nourishment of the hair and potential enhancement of hair strength and health.Nasya is an important Ayurvedic treatment for hair. It improves blood circulation, nourishes the hair, and promotes hair health. By delivering medicinal oils or herbs through the nose, Nasya helps address hair-related issues and strengthens the hair follicles. Regular Nasya can contribute to healthier and more vibrant hair.

As we all know consuming raw cow milk is the best way to get calcium and the worst part is in this generation many people are afraid of consuming good fat which is necessary for calcium absorption, so consuming good fat like nuts, ghee also helps

Note_in condition of lactose intolerance or inflammatory diesease You can maintain bone health without consuming milk by incorporating other calcium-rich foods in your diet like leafy greens, tofu, almonds, and sesame seeds. Additionally, getting enough vitamin D from sunlight exposure or supplements can also support bone health.

Note_ Almond nourishes all 7 dhatu or tissue of body, last tissue sukra semen takes months to get nourishment through food by almonds are best it instantly nourishes all tissues in the Body.

flaxseed can also be beneficial for reducing dandruff! The omega-3 fatty acids in flaxseed help nourish the scalp and reduce inflammation, which can contribute to dandruff. You can try massaging flaxseed oil onto your scalp or even mixing ground flaxseed with your shampoo for added benefits. Give it a try and see if it helps!

flaxseed is great for hair! It's rich in omega3 fatty acids, which can help promote healthy hair growth and reduce hair loss. You can try incorporating flaxseed oil or ground flaxseed into your diet or even use flaxseed oil as a hair mask. It's a natural and nourishing option for your hair To incorporate flaxseed into your haircare routine, you have a few options. One way is to use flaxseed oil as a hair mask. Simply apply it to your scalp and hair, leave it on for about 30 minutes, and then wash it out. Another option is to mix ground flaxseed with your favorite hair conditioner or styling product. This can help add extra nourishment to your hair. You can also consume flaxseed or flaxseed oil orally, as the omega-3 fatty acids can promote overall hair health. Give it a try and see how it works for you!

Roasted ground flaxseed with daal? That sounds like a tasty twist! Roasting flaxseeds can enhance their nutty flavor and add a crunchy texture. You can try roasting the ground flaxseed in a dry pan until it becomes fragrant and slightly golden, then sprinkle it on top of your daal for an extra burst of flavor and nutrition. It's a creative way to enjoy the benefits of flaxseed in your meal!

- In ayurveda it's said that low asthiagni(mitochondrial function of bone) cause bones, hair, nail, problem including discoloration of bones and teeth, spinal cord problems, toothache, all kinds of hair, nail and bones isse How to manage low mitochondrial function of bone in ayurveda consuming tikta/bitter herbs processed ghee or milk or taking basti a panchkarma therapy /Basti is a major panchakarma treatment used in Ayurveda. It involves the introduction of medicated oil, desi ghee, or herbal decoctions through the rectum.

  It helps eliminate toxic substances from the body, balances Vata dosha, and is beneficial in conditions like constipation, asthma, diabetes, hemorrhoids, and various digestive disorders.
- When calcium levels are low, it can disrupt the body's natural sleep-wake cycles. Calcium is involved in the regulation of neurotransmitters and hormones that play a role in sleep, such as melatonin. Low calcium levels may interfere with the production and release of these sleep-related substances, leading to difficulty falling asleep or

staying asleep at night and can cause stress, tension leading to hair fall,
It's important to maintain adequate calcium levels to support optimal sleep and hair.

- In Ayurveda, the "srotas" or channels are considered to be the pathways through which various substances flow in the body. The "savedvah srotas" specifically refer to the channels related to hair sweat pores and scalp health. It is believed that these channels are associated with the root of the hair, which in Ayurveda is associated with the "Vasa" or fat tissue and the "loomkup" or hair follicles. This nourishment plays a crucial role in maintaining the health and vitality of the hair.
- When the "savedvah srotas" (channels related to hair) are imbalanced, various factors can contribute to it. Excessive exercise, sunburn, consuming excessive cold foods, mental exertion, and emotions like anger, fear, and sadness can potentially disturb the balance of these channels. It is important to maintain a balanced lifestyle, including a healthy diet and managing emotions, to support the health of the hair and scalp.
  Steaming hair is believed to help open the pores on the scalp, which can enhance blood circulation and provide more nourishment to the hair follicles. This improved circulation can promote hair growth and contribute to healthier, stronger hair. Steaming can also help to moisturize and hydrate the hair, reducing dryness and improving its overall appearance.
  Steaming of hair in the postpartum period can have several benefits. It can help to stimulate blood circulation, promote hair growth, and provide nourishment to the scalp, which may help with

postpartum hair loss. Additionally, the steam can help to moisturize and hydrate the hair, making it more manageable and reducing dryness.

- Moisturizing the scalp twice a week is important because it helps maintain a healthy balance of moisture in the scalp and hair. This can prevent dryness, itchiness, and flakiness, which are common scalp issues. Moisturizing also nourishes the hair follicles, promoting healthy hair growth. It's like giving your scalp a refreshing drink of water to keep it hydrated and happy!
- Asatmaya food and food intolerance can lead to dusti or vikruti in the updhatu, which are the byproducts of the dhatu like hair, nails, ligaments, and so on. When we consume incompatible foods or foods that our body is intolerant to, it can disrupt the digestion and metabolism process, leading to imbalances in the tissues and byproducts. This can manifest as issues with hair, nails, ligaments, and other related structures. It's essential to maintain a healthy and balanced diet to support the proper nourishment and functioning of our body's tissue.food intolerances often involve digestive problems that are related to deficiencies in certain enzymes like lipase, pepsin, and amylase. These enzymes play crucial roles in breaking down fats, proteins, and carbohydrates during the digestive process. When there's a deficiency or imbalance in these enzymes, it can make it harder for the body to properly digest certain foods, leading to uncomfortable symptoms like bloating, gas, or stomach discomfort. Understanding your food intolerances and avoiding trigger foods can help manage these digestive issues.

- Raktaj krimi in Ayurveda is a condition caused by bloodborne parasites.When Raktaj krimi increases excessively, it can affect hair, nails, and eyelashes. It may lead to skin scavenging, weakening of ligaments, muscles, and cartilage. It is treated with herbal remedies and detoxification therapies.
- In Helminthic diseases, consuming pungent, bitter, astringent, alkalized, and warm herbs can be beneficial for blood cleansing. The qualities of pungent, bitter, astringent, alkaline, and warm herbs are opposite to Kapha, which helps in cleansing the blood. It's fascinating how Ayurveda utilizes these contrasting properties for the desired effect.
- Garlic, Tulsi (Holy Basil), mint, Raddish, Til (Sesame), and Vavding (Embelia ribes) are all beneficial herbs for cleansing the blood in cases of helminthic parasitic blood disorders. Ajmod (Celery seeds) is also known for its blood cleansing properties. Incorporating these herbs into your diet can be really beneficial.
- Applying warm ghee to the scalp in Ayurveda can help nourish the hair follicles, improve scalp health, and promote the growth of healthy tissues. Ghee is known for its moisturizing properties, which can help reduce dryness and support overall hair health. Try this treatment for better tissue scalp! in Ayurveda, warm ghee is sometimes used in non healing lesions It is believed that the application of warm ghee in specific areas can help balance the doshas and promote healing.
- For application on hair and scalp seed oil like sesame oil is very good because of it's penetrating power,

When it comes to seed oils for hair care, one option you can consider is using black seed oil. It's known for its potential benefits in promoting hair growth and reducing inflammation on the scalp.

- seed oil remedies for your hair, you can try using coconut oil or castor oil. They can help moisturize and strengthen your hair, promoting healthy growth. Just make sure to apply them to your hair and scalp, leave them on for a while, and then wash them out.
- Coconut oil and argan oil are known to penetrate the hair shaft better, providing deep hydration.
- Sesame oil can be used in various remedies for hair. One popular option is to mix sesame oil with a few drops of essential oils like lavender or rosemary, and then massage it into your scalp. Leave it on for a few hours or overnight before washing it out. This can help nourish your hair and promote a healthy scalp.
- In Ayurveda, there are various herbal remedies and treatments for hair health. One popular herb used for hair care is Amla (Indian gooseberry). It's believed to nourish the hair follicles, promote hair growth, and prevent premature graying. Other Ayurvedic remedies may include herbs like Brahmi, Bhringraj, and Neem.

Tips for haircare _ Trimming the hair regularly can help reduce hair fall by removing split ends and preventing breakage. When the ends of the hair are split, they can travel up the shaft and cause further damage, leading to increased hair fall. Trimming helps maintain the overall health of the hair, promoting stronger and less prone to breakage strands. However, it's important to note that trimming alone may not be a solution for underlying causes of hair fall, such as hormonal imbalances or nutrient deficiencies should be in check.

- Using grinded soapnut as a shampoo is an Ayurvedic practice that has been used for centuries. Soapnuts, also known as reetha or aritha, contain natural saponins that create a gentle lather when mixed with water. This lather helps cleanse the hair and scalp without stripping away natural oils.
- To use grinded soapnut as a shampoo, you can follow these steps:
- 1. Grind the soapnuts into a fine powder
- 2. Take a small amount of the powder or the soaked soapnuts and mix it with water to create a paste or lather.
- 3. Apply the paste or lather to wet hair and massage it into the scalp and hair.
- 4. Rinse thoroughly with water to remove the soapnut residue.
- Using soapnut as a shampoo can help remove dirt, excess oil, and product buildup from the hair. It is considered to be a natural and gentle alternative to commercial shampoos that may contain harsh chemicals.
- However, it's important to note that soapnut shampoo may not produce the same lather as regular shampoo, and it may take some time for your hair to adjust to this natural cleansing method.
- making hair oil using chopped onions and sesame oil. Here's a step-by-step guide:
- 1. Start by chopping an onion into small pieces.
- 2. Heat some sesame oil in a pan.

- 3. Add the chopped onion to the hot oil and let it cook until the oil turns black.
- 4. Once the oil has turned black, remove the pan from the heat and let the oil cool down for about 4 hours.
- 5. After the oil has cooled down, strain it to remove the onion particles.
- 6. Transfer the strained oil into a clean container or bottle.
- This homemade hair oil is believed to have nourishing properties and can be used to promote hair growth and improve overall hair health. However, it's important to note that results may vary for each individual. Eye care
- Indriya upghata _ eating less food
- Low levels of calcium and magnesium can contribute to weakness in the body and may also impact eye health. Calcium is essential for muscle function, including the muscles that support the eyes.

  Magnesium plays a role in nerve function and muscle relaxation, which can affect overall strength and eye health. It's important to maintain adequate levels of these minerals through a balanced diet or supplementation to support overall wellbeing and eye health.

- When calcium levels are low, it can disrupt the body's natural sleep-wake cycles. Calcium is involved in the regulation of neurotransmitters and hormones that play a role in sleep and muscle contraction, such as melatonin. Low calcium levels may interfere with the production and release of these sleeprelated substances, leading to difficulty falling asleep or staying asleep at night. It's important to maintain adequate calcium levels to support optimal sleep.

Dental health

Fluoride deficiency can contribute to an increased risk of developing teeth cavities. Fluoride helps strengthen tooth enamel and makes it more resistant to acid attacks from bacteria and sugars in the mouth. When there is a lack of fluoride, the enamel becomes weaker and more susceptible to decay, leading to the formation of cavities. It's important to ensure an adequate intake of fluoride through sources like fluoridated water, toothpaste, and dental treatments to help prevent tooth decay and maintain good oral health.

- To maintain a healthy fluoride level for your teeth, you can follow these tips:
    1. Use fluoride toothpaste: Brush your teeth twice a day with a fluoride toothpaste to help strengthen your tooth enamel.
    2. Drink fluoridated water: If your tap water contains fluoride, drink it regularly to help protect your teeth.
    3. Eat a balanced diet: Include foods and beverages that are good sources of fluoride, such as tea and fish, in your diet.

Ayurveda and dental care tips

- In Ayurveda, maintaining healthy teeth involves a holistic approach. Here are some Ayurvedic tips to support fluoride levels for healthy teeth:

1. Oil pulling: Swishing sesame oil or coconut oil in your mouth for a few minutes daily can help cleanse the mouth and support oral health.

2. Herbal tooth powders: Using herbal tooth powders made from ingredients like neem, clove, and licorice can help promote oral hygiene and maintain healthy teeth.
   Note _ better to buy dant manjan from any ayurvedic store
3. Ayurvedic diet: Consuming foods that are beneficial for oral health, such as fresh fruits, vegetables, and herbs like mint and turmeric, can support overall dental wellness.
4. Oral hygiene practices: Practicing proper oral hygiene, including regular brushing, flossing, and tongue cleaning, is essential for maintaining healthy teeth and gums.

- Remember, Ayurveda emphasizes individualized approaches, so it's always best to consult with an Ayurvedic practitioner for personalized guidance on maintaining fluoride levels and overall oral health. **Yogasan to promote better tooth care practicing yoga asanas that promote overall well-being and reduce stress can indirectly support dental health. Asanas like Sarvangasana (Shoulder Stand), Halasana (Plow Pose), and Matsyasana (Fish Pose) can improve blood circulation, reduce inflammation, and promote relaxation, which can be beneficial for oral health.**

Halasana, also known as the Plow Pose, is a yoga asana that involves lying on your back and lifting your legs over your head, aiming to touch your toes to the ground behind you. This asana helps stimulate the thyroid gland, improve digestion, and promote blood circulation to the head and neck area. While it may have some indirect benefits for oral health by improving overall circulation and reducing stress

- Sarvangasana, or the Shoulder Stand, is a yoga asana where you balance your body on your shoulders, with your legs extended vertically upwards. This asana is believed to improve blood circulation, boost metabolism, and promote overall well-being. While it may indirectly support dental health by improving blood flow to the head and neck region.
- Matsyasana, or the Fish Pose! It's a wonderful yoga asana where you lie on your back and arch your chest upward, resembling the graceful shape of a fish. This asana can help open up the chest, stretch the neck and shoulders, and improve posture. While it may not have direct benefits for tooth health or cavity prevention,
- Roar! Sihasana, or the Lion Pose, is a powerful yoga asana where you sit in a kneeling position, open your mouth wide, stick out your tongue, and roar like a lion. This asana helps release tension in the face and throat, and it's a great way to relieve stress and express your inner lion. While it may not have direct benefits for tooth health or cavity prevention, practicing Sihasana, along with maintaining good oral hygiene practices and regular dental check-ups, contributes to overall well-being. So go ahead, unleash your inner lion and let out a mighty roar.